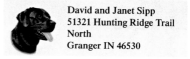

David and Janet Sipp
51321 Hunting Ridge Trail
North
Granger IN 46530

Stop Rising Healthcare Costs Using Toyota Lean Production Methods

38 Steps for Improvement

D1112013

Also available from ASQ Quality Press:

Lean-Six Sigma for Healthcare: A Senior Leader Guide to Improving Cost and Throughput
Chip Caldwell, Jim Brexler, and Tom Gillem

The Manager's Guide to Six Sigma in Healthcare: Practical Tips and Tools for Improvement
Robert Barry and Amy C. Smith

Nan: A Six Sigma Mystery
Robert Barry

Measuring Quality Improvement in Healthcare: A Guide to Statistical Process Control Applications
Raymond G. Carey, PhD and Robert C. Lloyd, PhD

The Six Sigma Book for Healthcare: Improving Outcomes By Reducing Errors
Robert Barry, PhD, Amy Murcko, APRN, and Clifford Brubaker, PhD

Improving Healthcare with Control Charts: Basic and Advanced SPC Methods and Case Studies
Raymond G. Carey

The Six Sigma Journey from Art to Science
Larry Walters

Six Sigma for the Office: A Pocket Guide
Roderick A. Munro

Defining and Analyzing a Business Process: A Six Sigma Pocket Guide
Jeffrey N. Lowenthal

Customer Centered Six Sigma: Linking Customers, Process Improvement, and Financial Results
Earl Naumann and Steven H. Hoisington

Office Kaizen: Transforming Office Operations into a Strategic Competitive Advantage
William Lareau

To request a complimentary catalog of ASQ Quality Press publications, call 800-248-1946, or visit our Web site at http://qualitypress.asq.org.

Stop Rising Healthcare Costs Using Toyota Lean Production Methods

38 Steps for Improvement

Robert Chalice

ASQ Quality Press
Milwaukee, Wisconsin

American Society for Quality, Quality Press, Milwaukee 53203
© 2005 by ASQ
All rights reserved. Published 2005
Printed in the United States of America

12 11 10 09 08 07 06 05   5 4 3 2 1

Library of Congress Cataloging-in-Publication Data

Chalice, Robert.
  Stop rising healthcare costs using Toyota lean production methods : 38
steps for improvement / Robert Chalice.
    p. cm.
  Includes bibliographical references and index.
  ISBN 0-87389-657-2 (soft cover, perfect bound : alk. paper)
  1. Medical care—United States—Cost control. 2. Medical care—United
States—Quality control. 3. Medical care—United States—Cost
effectiveness. 4. Production management—United States. 5. Production
control—United States. 6. Toyota Jidåosha Kabushiki
Kaisha—Management. I. Title.

  RA410.53.C43 2006
  362.1'0973—dc22   2005012649

ISBN 0-87389-657-2

Publisher: William A. Tony
Acquisitions Editor: Annemieke Hytinen
Project Editor: Paul O'Mara
Production Administrator: Randall Benson

ASQ Mission: The American Society for Quality advances individual,
organizational, and community excellence worldwide through learning,
quality improvement, and knowledge exchange.

Attention Bookstores, Wholesalers, Schools, and Corporations: ASQ Quality
Press books, videotapes, audiotapes, and software are available at quantity
discounts with bulk purchases for business, educational, or instructional use.
For information, please contact ASQ Quality Press at 800-248-1946, or write to
ASQ Quality Press, P.O. Box 3005, Milwaukee, WI 53201-3005.

To place orders or to request a free copy of the ASQ Quality Press Publications
Catalog, including ASQ membership information, call 800-248-1946. Visit our
Web site at www.asq.org or http://qualitypress.asq.org.

 Printed on acid-free paper

 Quality Press
600 N. Plankinton Avenue
Milwaukee, Wisconsin 53203
Call toll free 800-248-1946
Fax 414-272-1734
www.asq.org
http://qualitypress.asq.org
http://standardsgroup.asq.org
E-mail: authors@asq.org

Contents

Preface

What differentiates this book from other healthcare improvement books is that it is the only book currently available that presents a simple recipe of 38 lean steps for healthcare providers to reduce cost and improve quality. By following these straightforward steps, healthcare providers can adopt the same lean methods that have enabled companies like Toyota to become so successful.

This book has two teaching objectives. The reader will learn to:

1. Understand cost and quality issues facing healthcare in the United States.

2. Understand and implement a 38-step recipe to reduce healthcare costs and improve the quality of healthcare by using Toyota lean production methods.

Other books have presented Toyota's lean methods, but this book goes further by showing how to directly apply those successful methods to healthcare, where they are sorely needed.

Acknowledgments

Many thanks go to Jennifer Condel, Anatomic Pathology Team Leader, Dr. Stephen S. Raab, MD, David T. Sharbaugh, and Karen Wolk Feinstein, PhD at the University of Pittsburgh Medical Center Shadyside Hospital for an excellent lean case study in Appendix D entitled "Error-Free Pathology: Applying Lean Production Methods to Anatomic Pathology." A related article "Small Improvements Yield Big Results in Shadyside Pathology Lab" also appears in the August 2004 newsletter of the Pittsburgh Regional Healthcare Initiative (PRHI) Web site at http://prhi.org/newsletters.cfm. The online article was authored with the help of PRHI Communications Director Naida Grunden. The PRHI Web site at www.prhi.org contains numerous improvement examples that may be replicated by other healthcare providers. Contributors to the appendices are also credited within the appendices themselves.

I wish to thank Communications Director Naida Grunden, RN Team Leader Ellesha McCray and CEO Michael Moreland for "5S Catches on at the VA Pittsburgh Health System" in Appendix C.

I wish to thank Barb Bouché, Continuous Performance Improvement Manager at Seattle Children's Hospital and Regional Medical Center and others listed in the lean improvement example in Appendix B.

I wish to thank Mr. Dave LaCourse, IE, MS, for his past help, contributions, and encouragement. I wish to thank Paul Spaude, past president of Aspirus Health System (Wausau, Wisconsin) and current president of Borgess Health Alliance (Kalamazoo, Michigan), for his review of an early manuscript.

I wish to thank Paul O'Mara, Annemieke Hytinen, and Leayn and Paul Tabili for publishing assistance via ASQ Quality Press.

Finally I wish to thank my step mother and father, Eva and Walter, for their encouragement and guidance throughout my life, and my mother Mae for her nourishing love.

Part I

U.S. Healthcare System Problems and Solutions

1
U.S. Healthcare System Problems

RISING HEALTH INSURANCE PREMIUMS

Health coverage premiums rose at an annual rate of 11.2 percent in 2004 according to a survey of 2800 companies by the Kaiser Family Foundation done between January and May 2004. This is the fourth double-digit rise in the last four years. This compares to a 13.9 percent increase in 2003. In 2003, small firms experienced the largest increase in premiums, up 17 percent. If this trend continues, health coverage premiums will double again in about six years. By then, who will be able to afford it? Many companies with fewer than 25 employees have had to absorb premium increases of 25 percent or more this year. Think about what you now pay for health coverage. Then imagine yourself paying double that in possibly six years. This crisis is happening now. Figure 1.1 shows the year-to-year percentage change for health insurance premiums since 1988. The 2004 increase of 11.2 percent for health insurance premiums was approximately five times the general inflation rate of 2.3 percent, and five times the annual increase in worker earnings of about 2.2 percent. Over the last 20 years, health insurance premiums have increased annually on average at approximately three times the annual inflation rate.

In response, employers are shifting more and more healthcare costs to employees. Since 2000, the portion of the premium that employees pay has risen by nearly 50 percent. If you have the misfortune of

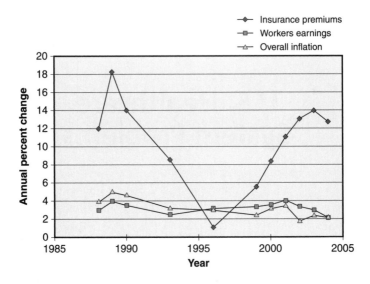

Figure 1.1   Year-to-year percentage change for health insurance premiums.

paying for your own health coverage, you are in an ever-tightening vise of increasing cost. Check out your own health insurance premium increases this year—up by 12 percent, 22 percent, or possibly even 40 percent! In 2002, my own personal group health insurance premium increased by 33 percent. In 2003, my premium increased again by 10 percent, and in 2004 it increased another 33 percent. My premium has nearly doubled in just three years, and I'm not alone. So the problem this book addresses is, "How do we stop these skyrocketing increases in healthcare costs?"[1]

W. Edwards Deming criticized excessive medical costs in the book *Four Days with Dr. Deming.*[2] Dr. Deming stated that his friend William Hoglund, who was manager of Pontiac Motor Division prior to 1995, told him, "Blue Cross is our second largest supplier. The cost of medical care is $400 per car." Six months later, Hoglund added that Blue Cross had overtaken steel as the most costly component in the automobile. That book was published over eight years ago, and with skyrocketing healthcare costs, the cost of healthcare in an automobile and all other U.S. products is no doubt much higher now. Some more recent data from a GM source in 2000 is as follows:

- GM spends $4.3 billion annually on healthcare.

- GM spends half as much on steel as it does on healthcare.

- Healthcare costs add about $1000 to the price of each GM product.

The $1000 cost for healthcare in each GM car in 2000 was about double what it was about six years earlier. It is clearly much higher now.

According to the United Auto Workers (UAW), "As of the second quarter of 2003, a UAW-represented assembler earns $25.63 per hour of straight time. A typical UAW-represented skilled-trades worker earns $29.75 per hour of straight time."[3] Appendix A shows that U.S. automobile manufacturers generally expend about 25 labor hours per manufactured vehicle. So if we use a worker's wage of $30 per hour times 25 hours per vehicle, the cost of labor in each vehicle is about $750. So, GM's cost for healthcare of $1000 per vehicle in 2000 is also significantly greater than its labor cost of $750 per vehicle. Healthcare cost per vehicle is now greater than either the cost of the steel or the workers' wages in each manufactured vehicle.

Consider again that automobile manufacturers now expend only about 25 hours of labor per each vehicle manufactured. That's rather astounding! These manufacturers can now make an entire automobile with just 25 hours of labor. That's because they have been continuously improving their processes, quality, and costs for years. Because of intense foreign competition, they either must improve or disappear. Healthcare can similarly follow their example to improve.

It is becoming increasingly difficult for American manufacturers to compete in world markets because of continually rising healthcare costs. Similarly, local school and city budgets have been hit hard by annual health insurance increases. Teacher counts and city services are being reduced to compensate for healthcare premium increases. For that matter, every purchaser of healthcare has been adversely affected.

Figure 1.2 illustrates changes in healthcare costs compared to other components of the Consumer Price Index (CPI) between 1990 and 2003. What we see is that the cost of hospital services, nursing home, and adult day care increased 2.4-fold from 1990 to 2003. If hospital service costs were presented alone without including nursing homes and adult day care, the increase would probably have been

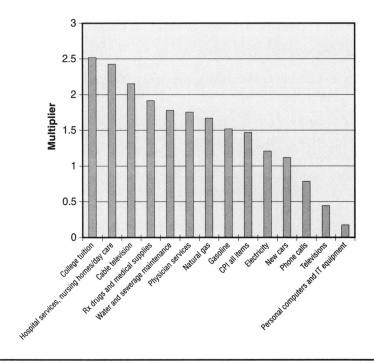

Figure 1.2 Cost in 2003 versus cost in 1990 (based on CPI data report).

much greater, possibly the highest on the graph. It is little comfort to see that only college tuition costs have had a greater increase. Also note that prescription drugs and medical supply costs increased 1.9-fold, while physician service costs increased 1.75 fold from 1990 to 2003. You usually hear people complain about continuing cost increases for cable TV, natural gas, gasoline, and electricity, but the fact is that hospital and other healthcare costs have outpaced them by a wide margin. Something has to be done to slow the steady rise of healthcare costs. That something is process improvement using lean production methods as described in this book. One consolation from the chart is that phone calls, televisions, and personal computers now cost you about half or less than what they cost in 1990. Unfortunately the costs for episodes of individual healthcare are also far greater in magnitude than most things on the chart. A hospital discharge might cost you $10,000 and it's increasing steadily. That's a lot more than a tank of gas or a monthly cable TV charge or home heating bill.[4]

WHY DOUBLE-DIGIT HEALTH INSURANCE INCREASES?

Why does the cost of health insurance coverage continue to increase at double-digit rates? Could it be that hospitals (and possibly physicians) generally represent near-monopolies in their service areas? If you're having a heart attack, are you going to question the cost of care at the nearest hospital?

Insured patients (governmental and commercially insured) comprise 85 percent of the U.S. population, and usually don't question healthcare charges even if they are exorbitant since their insurance will pay most of it. Their insurance softens the blow of exorbitant costs, even if their insurance premiums continually go up. How often do patients with insurance ask for the price of procedures beforehand? Not very often, because someone else is paying the bill. If every person was always spending only their own hard-earned dollars on their healthcare, there would be many more complaints.

Figure 1.3 shows a table from Lucette Lagnado's article "California Hospitals Open Books, Showing Huge Price Differences."[5]

How Much Is That Chest X-Ray?
A new California law allows patients to look up the retail prices of many goods and services at hospitals.
A survey of several hospital price lists shows dramatic differences in price.

	Scripps Memorial La Jolla, San Diego	Sutter General, Sacramento	UC Davis, Sacramento	San Francisco General, San Francisco	Doctors, Modesto	Cedars-Sinai Los Angeles	West Hills Hospital, West Hills
Chest X-ray (two views, basic)	$120.90	$790	$451.50	$120	$1,519	$412.90	$396.77
Complete blood count	$47	$234	$166	$50	$547.30	$165.80	$172.42
Comprehensive metabolic panel	$196.60	$743	$451**	$97	$1,732.95	$576	$387.18
CT-scan, head/brain (without contrast)	$881.90	$2,807	$2,868	$950	$6,599	$4,037.61	$2,474.95
Percocet* (or Crycodone hydrochloride and acetaminophen) one tablet, 5–325 mg	$11.44	$26.79	$15	$6.68	$35.50	$6.50	$27.86
Tylenol* (or acetaminophen) one tablet, 325 mg	$7.06	No charge	$1	$5.50	No charge	12 cents	$3.28

* Hospitals carry either generic version, name brand, or both
** Represents the added total of 14 tests that make up the comprehensive metabolic panel
Sources: Scripps Memorial, La Jolla; Sutter General; UC Davis Health System; San Francisco General; Doctors Medical Center; Cedars-Sinai Health System; West Hills Hospital and Medical Center

Figure 1.3 Huge hospital price variations.

A new law was enacted in California in 2004 that requires their hospitals to disclose the list prices of each patient chargeable item. Prior to this law, California hospitals, like nearly all other hospitals in the United States, kept their price lists secret. Patients generally had no idea of the gamut of charges they would face until they received their final bill. The new California law as well as initiatives in a few other states like Arizona, Wisconsin, and Minnesota are thankfully beginning to change this situation by opening hospitals' complete price lists. What is surprising is that these new disclosures show that prices can vary as much as 17-fold from one hospital to the next for the same item or service. The California table in Figure 1.3 shows for example that a "CT-scan of the head without contrast" varies from a low of $881 to a high of $6,599, a rather remarkable difference. What's bothersome is that these kinds of price variations are common when comparing random hospitals across the United States. This is a huge problem for consumers as well as the healthcare industry to address. Some semblance of rational pricing needs to prevail here. Admittedly, many patients do not pay list prices because they are part of an HMO or insurance group that has negotiated better pricing, or they are Medicare patients for whom the government pays a fixed amount based on their diagnosis and care episode. Unfortunately, the patients that are billed list prices are generally those without insurance who are the least able to pay since they have the least market clout. Lugnado's 12/27/04 *Wall Street Journal* article states "The elaborate pricing systems hospitals have developed over the years will be difficult to change, many in the industry say." Jan Emerson, spokeswoman for the California Healthcare Association adds "The entire system will have to be blown up." Clearly reform is needed here.

The healthcare union–sponsored organization Care of Ohio states "If you have no health insurance or your health insurance doesn't cover your bill, chances are you'll be expected to pay more than twice the price insured patients pay for the same treatment (see www.careforohio.org). Care for Ohio is a project launched by the members of SEIU District 1199, Ohio's healthcare union, to shine a light on the practices of hospitals. They make information available to patients, consumers, hospital employees, taxpayers, elected leaders, and community advocates to help promote the best decisions about healthcare—and make sure hospitals do their share to care for

Ohio." In March 2005, they published an outstanding report entitled "Twice the Price—What Uninsured and Under Insured Patients Pay for Hospital Care." They state "If health insurance doesn't cover your bill, you're in for a severe case of sticker shock." A billing system that charges twice as much to those who can least afford healthcare is clearly broken.[6]

Care of Ohio recommends:

> The ultimate solution, of course, is to create a healthcare system that guarantees everyone access to affordable healthcare. In the meantime, there are steps Ohio (and other states) can take to stop the overcharging of the uninsured, including: 1) Set limits on the prices hospitals can charge uninsured and underinsured patients, so that they will not be required to pay more for necessary medical care than it costs hospitals to provide it. 2) Create uniform charity care standards defining the amount of free and discounted care hospitals are expected to provide patients in need. 3) Require far greater transparency and disclosure so that Ohio (and other) hospitals make their prices more accessible to consumers, publicize the availability of charity care, and report to the state annually the number and income of self-paying patients, the prices charged and free care provided, and the actual cost of providing the care.

Although Care of Ohio recommendations are important, they do not reduce the fundamental existing waste and inefficiency in related healthcare processes. It's important to go beyond their recommendations to improve the care delivery processes themselves by eliminating all forms of waste.

When there is more than one healthcare provider in a service area, how much duplicate technology and facilities are there and how much does that add to the overall cost of healthcare? As an example, the Honorable David Durenberger, U.S. Senate (R-MN, 1978 to 1995), noted in a 2005 presentation that there are 21 CT scanners within 2.1 miles of Fairview Southdale Hospital near Minneapolis, Minnesota. Is that rational from a cost perspective, or does it reflect a healthcare system that is simply out of control?

Healthcare providers operate by their own nature in a survival mode. Each is trying to overcome the other in a race for market share, growth, and dominance. Competing providers do not generally operate in a synergistic manner to complement one another. Their goal is to simply capture and maintain market share. Shouldn't their goal instead be to achieve the best healthcare status at the lowest cost for the entire population of a region?

For years, as shown in Figure 1.1, healthcare providers chose to increase costs rather than embrace lean delivery methods to lower costs or even keep costs the same from year to year. At the same time, providers continually try to increase prices and profits, to the extent that employers and the public will endure. Some healthcare administrators have personally told me they are concerned that reducing costs may cause the patient to perceive that they are receiving lower quality care. It makes one wonder what will indeed motivate hospital administrators to lower costs. They don't seem to do it voluntarily. If a healthcare provider embraced lean methods to lower cost, that would indeed force other competing providers to slowly follow suit. According to the Wisconsin Hospital Association (WHA), the reasons for escalating costs include:

Advances in patient care. Advances in medical treatments and technologies mean higher survival rates and safer, more convenient hospital services. These advances are costly to fund.

Input costs. Workforce shortages are driving up healthcare worker salaries at rates much higher than inflation.

Government underfunding. The Medicare and Medicaid programs *dramatically* underpay their fair share of hospital expenses, forcing hospitals to shift costs to private payers.

Employer-sponsored health insurance. Lack of economic consequences for employees leads to higher consumption.

Less than optimum care. The Midwest Business Group on Health (MBGH) says 30 percent of the cost of care is due to poor quality.

45 MILLION AMERICANS ARE
WITHOUT HEALTH INSURANCE

In 2003, the number of Americans without health insurance rose by 1.4 million to 45 million, or 15.6 percent of the population.[7]

That's more than the combined population of the nation's 24 smallest states plus the District of Columbia. It's also about 1.25 times the entire population of California, the largest state in the United States. Imagine all the people in California being far less than the total uninsured in the United States. In August 2004, the U.S. Census Bureau released figures showing that 15.6 percent of Americans were uninsured during 2003 compared to 15.2 percent in 2002, and 14.6 percent in 2001.[5] This increasing trend in the number of uninsured is ominous. In 2003, there was an increase of 1.5 million uninsured compared to a 2.4 million increase in 2002. The total increase of 3.9 million uninsured in 2002 and 2003 is larger than the population of either metropolitan Los Angeles or Chicago, which are the second and third largest cities in the United States, exceeded only by the population of metropolitan New York. Understand that the group of uninsured in the United States actually grew in 2002 and 2003 by an amount larger than metropolitan Los Angeles's population! More than one in seven U.S. citizens did not have health insurance coverage during 2003.

The rising cost of healthcare coverage is contributing to the growing crisis of the uninsured in the United States. In 2003, the percentage of people covered by employer-based health insurance fell to 60.4 percent from 61.3 percent the year before, no doubt again because more could not afford it.

In the United States it is a right of each citizen to receive a public education through high school. Should it not also be a right of each U.S. citizen to receive affordable health insurance and affordable healthcare? The CEO of a large U.S. healthcare system once commented to me that when he looked at the list of personal bankruptcies frequently published in the local newspaper, he observed that the majority were due to healthcare-related bills. In 2005, a Harvard study concluded that half of all U.S. bankruptcy filers stated that medical expenses led to their financial downfall and most of them had health insurance.[8] They also found a 30-fold increase in medically related bankruptcies compared to a similar study conducted in 1981.

Medical bankruptcies affect up to 2.2 million Americans.[9] Isn't it time that we, as a nation, provide our citizens with a basic level of healthcare so that major illnesses don't leave them destitute?

MOTIVATING HEALTHCARE PROVIDERS TO REDUCE COST AND IMPROVE QUALITY

An important question is, what will motivate healthcare providers, particularly hospitals, to truly embrace high-quality, lean production methods? As long as patients and employers continue to accept and endure continually rising healthcare premiums and costs, there is little hope. When the cost of healthcare becomes so outrageous that individuals and employers can no longer afford it, then change may occur as they clamor loudly. After the cost of healthcare doubles again, picket lines may appear in front of healthcare facilities and insurers. This may come to pass within the next six years, as healthcare costs are projected to double again if the current trend continues. A few future scenarios are possible: (1) public and employer outrage will produce meaningful voluntary cost reduction; (2) partial government intervention (and cost control) will occur; or (3) the U.S. healthcare system will be nationalized as it is in many other countries (for example, Canada). While some may argue against nationalized healthcare in the United States, nearly everyone agrees that U.S. healthcare has become just too expensive. To date, healthcare providers and insurers have not held down or reduced costs on their own. Healthcare costs are presently rising at about five times the rate of overall inflation (see Figure 1.1). Few, if any, would disagree with the objective of simply reducing U.S. healthcare costs.

One may ask why healthcare providers have not yet embraced lean methods as other U.S. manufacturers have. To be frank, many healthcare providers are near-monopolies in their service areas. They have had little reason to embrace lean. By comparison, a manufacturer with increasingly low-cost foreign competition from China, Asia, or Mexico has been forced to embrace lean or become extinct.

Healthcare worker shortages may encourage providers to embrace lean methods to be more efficient with limited available talent. From

2000 to 2010, employment in healthcare occupations is expected to grow 29 percent, or more than twice the 14 percent growth rate of non-healthcare jobs. During that 10-year period, job growth of between 45 percent to 62 percent is expected for personal care aides, medical assistants, physician assistants, medical record technicians, home health aides, physical and occupational therapy aides and assistants, and audiologists.[10] Corresponding healthcare worker shortages may encourage providers to slowly embrace lean methods.

The 2004 report "Manufacturing in America—A Comprehensive Strategy to Address the Challenges to U.S. Manufacturers" by the U.S. Department of Commerce *lists reducing healthcare costs as a number one priority.*[11]

Between 2000 and 2003, the United States lost 15.1 percent or 2.6 million of its manufacturing jobs. The report states, "The challenges confronting American manufacturers and manufacturing workers are urgent, and President Bush has already taken action. He has implemented a jobs and growth agenda and outlined a six-point plan." Note that the number one priority is to reduce healthcare costs.

1. To make healthcare costs more affordable.

2. To reduce the lawsuit burden on the U.S. economy.

3. To ensure an affordable, reliable energy supply.

4. To streamline regulations and reporting requirements.

5. To open markets for American products.

6. To enable families and businesses to plan for the future with confidence.

Keith Guggenberger of Starkey Labs summed up the perspective of many U.S. manufacturers at a roundtable in Minneapolis, "Healthcare is a big part of the concerns of policy that we have in keeping us competitive. At Starkey, we spend almost $8000 per employee on healthcare in the U.S., and when half of our people make under $28,000 a year, it is hard to make those sorts of ends meet. The rising cost of healthcare is the biggest barrier to health coverage. The annual family health insurance premium increased to $9068 in spring 2003." Note that the family healthcare premium is equal to almost one-third of the employee's salary. What these facts suggest is that there is economic and competitive value for reducing the growth in healthcare costs that U.S. manufacturing companies face, particularly for small and medium-sized manufacturers that are the foundation of the U.S. manufacturing sector.

What's in it for hospital administrators who embrace lean? To date they haven't done so voluntarily. This is a pivotal point. If there isn't enough incentive to promote positive change, healthcare leaders and their organizations will adhere to the status quo of increasing costs with marginal quality. Healthcare leaders may not be experiencing the kind of "burning platform" that forced most U.S. manufacturers to embrace lean to simply survive amidst growing Chinese, Mexican, and Asian competition. If they would embrace a lean system, hospital administrators would:

- Produce meaningful cost and quality improvement.

- Achieve strategic advantage over competition.

- Quell growing business and public clamoring about healthcare costs.

- Earn greater prestige and national recognition.

- Generate greater profit.

- Provide money for uninsured, uncompensated care and philanthropy.

- Help fend off government intervention, cost control, and nationalized healthcare.

- Better utilize increasingly scarce healthcare workers.

These points may not be adequate to propel administrators to embrace lean. Hospitals in particular do not generally face severe enough economic consequences to force them to adopt lean methods. If they do not, government intervention may be unavoidable.

TOYOTA LEAN PRODUCTION

To solve the problems of rising healthcare costs and questionable quality, we will turn to the techniques used by one of the most successful automobile companies in the world, the Toyota Motor Company. On May 5, 2003, the *Detroit News* published an article entitled "Profit-Rich Toyota Threatens Big Three—Can Anything Stop Toyota?" Toyota reported net profits of roughly $10.2 billion for its last fiscal year ending 3/31/04. That was more than any Detroit automaker has made in any one year since at least the 1960s and more than GM, Ford, and Chrysler combined made in 2004. Realize that Toyota was nearly bankrupt in 1949 and then terminated a large part of its workforce.

By implementing what has become known as the Toyota Lean Production System (TPS), Toyota has become the de facto standard by which American automobile executives judge their own companies. Compared to traditional mass production techniques, Toyota manufactures with half the human effort in the factory, half the manufacturing space, half the investment tools, half the engineering hours, and half the time to develop new products. Despite being the most efficient car maker in the world, Toyota produces "world-class quality" automobiles. In the June 2004 "J.D. Power Dependability Study," Toyota captured the best dependability rankings with seven models topping their vehicle classes. Toyota also has the highest customer retention rate in the automobile industry. That is, a higher percentage of Toyota owners repurchase another Toyota, as compared to any other automobile brand.

Similarly, the April 2005 "Consumer Reports Reliability Study" ranks 10 Japanese models "most reliable" with no U.S. domestic models in the top 10. The April 2005 *Consumer Reports* "Quick Picks" of 82 best cars based on high ratings, reliability, fuel economy, safety, and overall satisfaction includes no U.S. domestic models. This issue also lists 32 cars that greater than 80 percent would "purchase again"—that list contains 25 Japanese models dominated by Toyota and only one U.S. model, the Chevrolet Corvette. The remainder are European luxury sedans and sports cars.

Toyota uses TPS to deliver best quality, lowest cost, and shortest product manufacturing time through the incessant elimination of waste. Toyota focuses on the tasks and responsibilities of those workers who actually add value to the car and reduces or eliminates all other non-value-added tasks and labor. TPS is comprised of three pillars: just-in-time production with just-in-time inventory, built-in quality at each step without the need for reinspection, and respect for the employee. *Quality* is defined as "meeting or exceeding customer expectations." Alternatively, it may be defined as "meeting or exceeded predefined standards." Either definition is workable and interchangeable. Clearly, American industry and, by extension, the U.S. healthcare system, has much to learn from Toyota's efficient yet high-quality methods.

The Lean Enterprise Institute[12] defines *lean production* as:

A business system for organizing and managing product (or service) development, operations, suppliers, and customer (patient) relations that requires less human effort, less space, less capital, and less time to make products (services) with fewer defects to precise customer desires, compared with the previous system.

Lean production was pioneered by Toyota after World War II and, as of 1990, typically required half the human effort, half the manufacturing space and capital investment for a given amount of capacity, and a fraction of the development and lead time of mass production systems, while making products in wider variety at lower volumes with many fewer defects. The term was coined by John Krafcik, a research assistant at MIT with the International Motor Vehicle Program in the late 1980s.

Lean thinking is a five-step thought process proposed by James Womack and Dan Jones in their 1996 book *Lean Thinking* to guide managers through a lean transformation.[13] The steps are:

1. Specify value from the standpoint of the end customer.

2. Identify all the steps in the value stream.

3. Make the value creating steps flow toward the customer.

4. Let customers pull value (toward them) from the next upstream activity.

5. Pursue perfection.

WASTE IN HEALTHCARE

Don Berwick, president and CEO of the Institute for Healthcare Improvement (IHI), estimates that 30 percent to 40 percent of the total cost of healthcare production is waste or as the Japanese call it, *muda.* Cindy Jimmerson, a nurse who has also been pursuing lean healthcare methods, states, "The national numbers for waste in healthcare are between 30 percent and 40 percent, but the reality of what we've observed doing minute-by-minute observation over the last three years is closer to 60 percent. That's waste of time, waste of money, waste of material resources. It's nasty. The waste is not limited to administrative costs, which most research on healthcare has documented. It's everywhere: patient care and non–patient care alike." Jim Womack, founder of the Lean Enterprise Institute, similarly estimates that organizations can generally save 50 percent of labor and space by converting to lean production methods similar to Toyota's.

Is it possible that our healthcare delivery system can similarly save 50 percent by converting to lean production? By *lean production* I mean the elimination of waste in all its forms, whether time, materials, or unneeded process steps. By *lean processes* I don't mean making employees work harder. I do mean eliminating all waste and non-value-added steps in work processes to improve cost and quality.

The healthcare industry itself has much to gain by adopting Toyota's lean methods to reduce cost and improve quality, as I will further present. What's most critical is for U.S. healthcare executives to embed into their organizations a mindset of continuous cost and quality improvement. This means setting a goal that there will be no cost (or insurance premium) increase this year for patients. Even better, healthcare executives should say, "There will be an X percent cost reduction, and we will simultaneously achieve quality improvement goals, and specific community health objectives."

Cost per case mix indexed (CMI) adjusted patient discharge is defined as the cost per discharged patient adjusted for patient severity. It is a comparable cost indicator across all hospitals. Why is there such huge variability in cost per CMI-adjusted discharge across the country, from around $5000 at the lowest-cost hospitals to possibly more than $15,000 per discharge at the highest-cost hospitals? You may pay a different price for the same hospital stay or medical procedure all across the country. There is little consistency in the actual price and quality of medical care across the United States.

Remember our precept that the treatment of a patient is primarily between them and their physician and nurse(s) and supporting ancillary departments. Yet large administrative support structures exist around the physicians and nurses and critical supporting departments. Thirty-one cents of every dollar spent for healthcare in the United States goes to administrative costs, according to an August 20, 2003 article in the *New England Journal of Medicine*.[14] That's nearly double the rate in Canada. According to that article, the United States spent $294 billion on healthcare paperwork and administration in 1999. Having a delivery system in the United States administered as efficiently as the one in Canada would save $209 billion annually, the authors say, enough to insure all Americans who now lack health insurance.

It's clear that there are plenty of opportunities to reduce healthcare costs in the United States. In this book, hospital executives can learn how Toyota lean production works and how to apply it to their organizations to continuously lower cost and improve quality to reach board approved goals.[15]

In addition to Canada, other countries that have a good, successful single-payer system in place include France, Germany, and Holland. These single-payer systems standardize all the paperwork, greatly reduce administrative costs, eliminate the underwriting and health insurance application process, eliminate the patient payment process as they are funded by increased taxes, and provide a defined level of healthcare to each citizen. In 2003, Maine became the first U.S. state to enact a single-payer health system for every Maine resident. It is projected to save $1 billion by 2008, compared to Maine's 2004 health expenditures of $8.4 billion. The Maine system will also be able to negotiate statewide for better pharmaceutical prices. And, Maine plans to penalize pharmaceutical companies that refuse to sell drugs to uninsured people at the same discounted prices that Medicaid pays.

Streamlining payer methods will help reduce administrative waste, but this does *nothing* to attack the other root cause, wasteful healthcare operating practices.

U.S. HEALTH EXPENDITURES ARE A GROWING PERCENTAGE OF GDP

According to the government-run Center for Medicare and Medicaid Services, total national personal healthcare expenditures were $1.3 trillion in calendar year 2000, or nearly 14 percent of gross domestic product (GDP).[16] Of that total, $412 billion (32 percent) were for hospital services, $286 billion (22 percent) for physician services, $122 billion (9 percent) for prescriptions, and $92 billion (7 percent) for nursing home service. Hospitals account for the greatest percent by far (32 percent) of total national healthcare expenditures, nearly 1.5 times total physician expense. Hospitals are the top priority, but all healthcare providers, including physician practices, pharmaceutical companies, and nursing homes, are candidates for lean improvements. Between 2001 and 2011, health spending is projected to grow 2.5 percent per year faster than the GDP, so that it will constitute 17 percent of the GDP within the next seven years. (See Figure 1.4). It is interesting to note that France and Italy were ranked number one and two in health system effectiveness by the World Health Organization, and they each spend only 8 percent to 10 percent of their GPD on healthcare.[17] It is also interesting that Italy, which

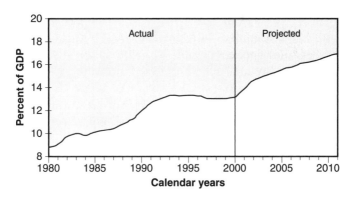

Figure 1.4   National health expenditures as a share of gross domestic product (GDP). Between 2001 and 2011, health spending is projected to grow 2.5 percent per year faster than GDP, so that by 2011 it will constitute 17 percent of GDP.

has the third largest health system in Europe, behind Germany and France, spends 41 percent of its health expenditures on physicians, 18 percent on hospital care, and 11 percent on drugs. While drug expenditures are similar percentagewise to the 9 percent of GDP spent in the United States, Italy spends far less on hospital care—18 percent of the GDP compared to 32 percent in the United States, or almost half as much. This is consistent with a lean goal of saving one half. Conversely, Italy spends almost twice as much on physicians, 41 percent of GDP compared to 22 percent in the United States. Back to our premise that a patient's care is primarily between them and their physician and nurse(s), Italy's greater proportion of funding for physicians makes sense since physicians usually provide patient value-added services.

A March 2004 headline in *USA Today* reads, "Medicare System Projected to Go Broke in 15 Years." This would be 2019, which is seven years earlier than previously predicted.[18]

A current report from the trustees of Medicare and Social Security blames this deterioration on "lower-than-expected revenue from workers' payroll taxes, higher spending on healthcare, and the prescription drug benefit Congress passed in 2003." The report shows that the expenses for Medicare will exceed the revenue from payroll taxes and beneficiary premiums as soon as 2011, which is less than six years from now. Clearly, some important changes are needed to reduce the cost of healthcare, reduce Medicare expenses, and/or increase Medicare funding.

THE UNITED STATES RANKS 37th IN HEALTH SYSTEM PERFORMANCE

The United States spends more than any other country per capita on healthcare. The United States spends per capita on healthcare nearly twice as much as each of the next highest spending countries of Switzerland, Norway, Germany, and Canada.[19] See Figures 1.5, 1.6, and 1.7. At the same time that U.S. health expenditures and insurance premiums continue rising at unprecedented rates, the quality of U.S. healthcare remains a serious issue. We're paying more, but not necessarily getting better quality. According to a study by the World Health Organization done in 2000, the United States ranked 37th in

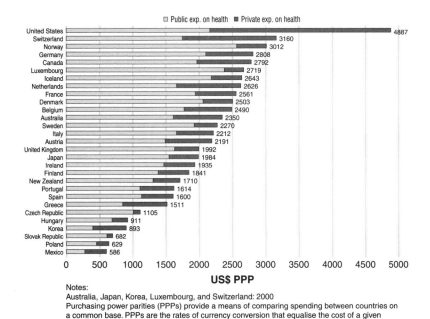

Figure 1.5 Health expenditure per capita, US$ PPP, 2001.

Source: OECD Health Data 2003.

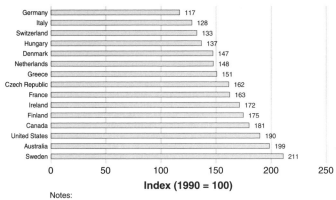

Figure 1.6 Growth in pharmaceutical expenditure per capita, in real terms, 1990–2001 (1990 = 100).

Source: OECD Health Data 2003.

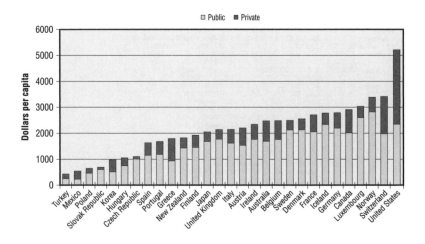

Figure 1.7   Public and private expenditure on health, U.S. dollars per capita, calculated using purchasing power parities (PPPs), 2002.

the world out of 191 countries in health system performance, with France and Italy ranking first and second, even though they spend half as much per capita on healthcare. Based on key national performance indicators, healthcare in the United States is not as cost effective as in 36 other countries. Also, U.S. pharmaceutical charges are increasing at the third fastest rate within Organization for Economic Cooperation and Development countries even though most pharmaceutical companies are located in the United States. See Figure 1.6. Surprisingly, the United States ranked 26th among industrialized countries for infant mortality rates, with 7.2 deaths per 1000 live births or .72 percent. This is nearly double the rate in Sweden, Finland, Norway, and Japan.[20]

QUALITY PROBLEMS IN U.S. HEALTHCARE

The Chicago-based Midwest Business Group on Health was founded in January 1980 by a group of Midwestern employers to address a common problem—escalating healthcare costs that threatened the competitiveness of U.S. employers and the welfare of their employees, families, and the population at large.[21] The organization estimates that 30 percent of total U.S. healthcare costs result from poor quality. This estimate is consistent with lean producers' claims to improve efficiency by 50 percent by removing waste and streamlining processes. The group's definition of poor-quality healthcare is shown in Figure 1.8.

According to a study published in the *New England Journal of Medicine* in 2003, participating patients received only 54.9 percent of recommended care.[22] Based on this study, it is little different than a coin toss as to whether a patient will receive recommended care for a given condition. The study involved telephoning a random sample of 13,275 adults in 12 metropolitan areas and asking them about their selected healthcare experiences. Investigators also received written consent to copy medical records for the most recent two-year period to evaluate performance based on 439 indicators of quality of care for 30 acute and chronic conditions as well as preventive care. Quality varied markedly by medical condition, ranging from a high of 78.7 percent of recommended care delivered for senile cataract to a low of 10.5 percent of recommended care delivered for alcohol dependence. This study concludes, "The deficits we have identified in adherence to recommended processes for basic care pose serious

MBGH definition of poor quality includes:

- *Overuse.* A variety of surgical procedures, tests, medications, and treatments are overused, driving up costs unnecessarily while simultaneously exposing patients to risks of complication and sometimes even death.

- *Underuse.* Providers routinely fail to administer a variety of known-to-be-effective tests and treatments to heart attack victims and individuals with diabetes and congestive heart failure.

- *Misuse.* Medical errors represent the most common form of misuse within the healthcare system, with drug misuse representing the most frequent form of error.

- *Waste.* Waste, primarily in the form of unnecessary administrative activities, is prevalent throughout healthcare, as it is in many other industries.

Figure 1.8   The Midwest Business Group on Health estimates 30 percent of total costs results from poor-quality healthcare.

threats to the health of the American public. Strategies to reduce these deficits in care are warranted." This study provides strong support for better standardizing care processes just as Toyota standardized its manufacturing process steps.

In its November 1999 report, "To Err Is Human: Building a Safer Health System," the Institute of Medicine states:

> Healthcare in the United States is not as safe as it should be—and can be. At least 44,000 people, and perhaps as many as 98,000 people, die in hospitals each year as a result of medical errors that could have been prevented, according to estimates from two major studies. The knowledgeable health reporter for the *Boston Globe*, Betsy Lehman, died from an overdose during chemotherapy. Willie King had the wrong leg amputated. Ben Kolb was eight years old when he died during 'minor' surgery due to a drug mix-up.

These horrific cases that make the headlines are just the tip of the iceberg. Two large studies, one conducted in Colorado and Utah and the other in New York, found that adverse events occurred in 2.9 percent and 3.7 percent of hospitalizations, respectively. That is, approximately one in 21 patients experiences an adverse event during their hospitalization. The study in Colorado and Utah implies that at least 44,000 Americans die each year as a result of medical errors. The New York study suggests the number of deaths may be as high as 98,000.

Even when using the lower estimate, U.S. deaths due to medical errors represent the seventh leading cause of death in the United States. More people die in a given year as a result of medical errors than from motor vehicle accidents (43,458), breast cancer (42,297), or AIDS (16,516). Only a few hundred people die each year from airplane crashes. Think about that. *The seventh leading cause of deaths in the United States is medical errors.* Much more effort needs to be focused on reducing this horrendous statistic.

> *Medical errors* can be defined as the failure of a planned action to be completed as intended or the use of a wrong plan to achieve an aim. Among the problems that commonly occur during the course of providing healthcare are adverse drug events and improper transfusions, surgical injuries and

wrong-site surgery, suicides, restraint-related injuries or death, falls, burns, pressure ulcers, and mistaken patient identities. High error rates with serious consequences are most likely to occur in intensive care units, operating rooms, and emergency departments. Beyond their cost in human lives, preventable medical errors exact other significant tolls. They have been estimated to result in total costs (including the expense of additional care necessitated by the errors, lost income and household productivity, and disability) of between $17 billion and $29 billion per year in hospitals nationwide.

It is not sufficient to address excessive medical errors by just adding more staff and more costs. Rather it is important to get at the root causes of errors and to design systems that make the errors impossible to occur.

Healthcare providers need to adopt an important technique from the aerospace industry called failure mode and effects analysis (FMEA) to reduce errors in healthcare. FMEA originated in the 1960s to improve safety in the aerospace and chemical industries. The goal of FMEA is to prevent safety accidents from ever occurring. This is precisely what we wish to accomplish within healthcare. The automotive and other industries have similarly adopted FMEA analyses, and it's time for the healthcare industry to do likewise. The simple FMEA technique can help reduce the 98,000 medically related deaths and billions is unnecessary costs annually.[23]

The steps within an FMEA analysis are shown in column 5 of Table 3.1, page 50. FMEA can be a simple process, as follows:

a. Perform a detailed review of the product or process. A team may be used.

b. Brainstorm all ways the process can fail, that is, all failure modes.

c. List the potential effects of each failure mode.

d. Assign a 1–10 *severity* rating for each effect. 10 = highest.

e. Assign a 1–10 probability of *occurrence* rating for each failure mode. 10 = highest probability.

 f. Assign a 1–10 *detection* rating for each failure mode and/or effect. 10 = not detectable.

 g. Calculate the risk priority number (RPN) for each effect (= severity# × occurrence# × detection#). Add them all together to get the total RPN for all effects related to a given failure mode.

 h. Prioritize the failure modes for action via RPN score (that is, list the failure modes in decreasing order by RPN score).

 i. Take action to eliminate or reduce the high RPN failure modes.

 j. Calculate the resulting RPN as the failure modes are reduced or eliminated. These new RPN scores should be zero or at least now greatly reduced.

FAILURE OF CONTINUOUS QUALITY IMPROVEMENT AND TOTAL QUALITY MANAGEMENT

Continuous quality improvement (CQI) is a process of continuously making everything better each day. It is customer focused and requires that processes be analyzed, measured, and improved on an ongoing basis. It has essentially failed in healthcare in the past because it was not implemented widely or continuously throughout the organization. Rather, it occurs sporadically every four years just before inspections by the Joint Commission for Accreditation of Healthcare Organizations (JCAHO). CQI has not generally been pervasive and continuous within healthcare organizations and it has basically failed to markedly improve overall cost and quality. It has not involved most employees and rarely has been focused on cost in healthcare.

 Total quality management (TQM) is a management system in which everyone within an organization constantly monitors what they do to find ways to improve quality of operations, products, services, marketing, customer and employee satisfaction, and everything else about the organization. It is a broader concept that includes CQI. Every individual is responsible for improving the quality of goods and services supplied. Ford with its "Quality is job one" slogan illustrates this organizationwide philosophy. TQM has basically failed in healthcare organizations as most employees simply didn't understand it. Like CQI, it has not been pervasive throughout organizations and has been intermittently applied. It too has rarely been focused on cost in healthcare.

Basically, CQI and TQM approaches were implemented to satisfy JCAHO requirements and have not moved healthcare organizations toward world-class levels of low cost and high quality. CQI and TQM have not generally been the primary focus of hospital boards. A new approach is needed where hospital boards, administrators, and all staff continuously focus on improving healthcare cost and quality. For this to occur, they must receive adequate rewards and/or negative consequences or the status quo will reign or worse, degenerate.

REDESIGNING THE U.S. HEALTHCARE SYSTEM

If a reasonable person were to redesign a new U.S. healthcare system from scratch, they would not likely come up with anything like the U.S. healthcare system (or should we say nonsystem) that we have today. The system we have today has evolved over the last two hundred years or so from its beginnings as a cottage industry. Each early healthcare provider grew independently within a generally noncoordinated system of similar healthcare providers that has become more like a patchwork quilt than a designed system.

If designed in a logical manner, each healthcare provider would currently serve a certain-sized population in a certain geographic area without duplication. Smaller satellite centers would refer patients to larger centers to address more difficult cases. The most difficult cases would be addressed by regional and national centers with extensive capabilities and specialty expertise. A logically designed national healthcare system would look more like a tree with satellite centers as its small branches, regional centers as its large branches, and national centers as its trunk. All costs and charges would be uniform across the United States except for small cost-of-living adjustments.

Possibly there should be a law that all hospital charges be equal to the appropriate Medicare charge plus X percent. In fact, the Medical Savings Insurance Company of Oklahoma recently filed a lawsuit against certain Florida hospitals that were refusing to accept its routine payments of Medicare charges plus 20 percent for treatment of any non-Medicare patients.[24]

In a well-designed system, all patients would also have uniform access to services, and duplication would be minimized within each service area. In a move in this direction, some states now require a hospital to complete a certificate of need before new construction is approved. This is not, however, required in many states. At minimum, our government should institute a national certificate of need process for all healthcare providers to make services uniformly available across the nation and evenly distribute costs. Our current system, which has run amok, is more like a garden that is overgrown with a variety of plants and weeds. Each plant and weed continually tries to overtake the other in an uncontrolled, erratic manner. What determines which one survives and grows is more a matter of the strength of warring factions than any logical design to achieve specific community goals of cost and quality.[25]

The United States will sooner or later need to coordinate its current nonsystem of healthcare. A national imperative is for our country to create a target design for an ideal healthcare delivery system and to create incentives for all stakeholders to begin to gradually move from our current nonsystem toward that ideal design. Maybe it's time to create a new, spartan, but highly functional, hospital design that provides good nurse staffing; good access to competent physician(s) who attend to patients; and good ancillary lab, x-ray, and pharmacy services, all contained in a compact, low-cost facility that eliminates all the other services that a patient does not wish to personally pay for. Maybe it's time to construct a hospital model that is simply centered on the patient, their physician, their nurses, and critical ancillary functions, and that contains little or no excess overhead. This ideally designed healthcare system would also minimize handoffs of the patient among too many different physicians and hospital staff. How can a patient receive quality care if too many participants are involved who aren't comparing notes? A similar streamlined, spartan design also may be considered for any other type of health care provider.

2

Respect for Employees

The immediate key to stopping the rise in healthcare costs is to eliminate all forms of waste in healthcare. This can be started now without the need for any new legislation. However, wholesale reengineering or downsizing efforts create extreme ill will and must be avoided at all costs. It is critical for hospital administrators to create an environment of trust and honesty, employee community, and mutual respect.

W. Edwards Deming aptly stated as one of his quality improvement principles, "Drive out fear, build trust." Deming also stated that 80 percent of problems are management or system related. Similarly, Taiichi Ohno, father of TPS, focuses on "respect for humanity" as one of his guiding principles for building a lean, low-cost, high-quality production system. Peter Drucker also contends that each organization has a major goal of personal growth for its employees.

After World War II, Japan historically tried to maintain long-term employment (lifetime employment) for core personnel, whose experiences were important assets to Japanese companies. We should show the same high ethical standards toward all employees while rebuilding the U.S. healthcare system into a lean, low-cost, high-quality system. It's important to base management decisions on a long-term view of developing and retaining dedicated and valuable employees, even at the expense of short-term financial goals. Promote the concept of the "family of employees" with its members truly receiving earned respect. These employees will then commit long-term to providing truly value-added services to patients and customers. Grow leaders and high-performing employees from within who are committed to the organization.

Michael Hammer, the renowned reengineering expert, stated in one of his reengineering training videos that the "soft stuff" is "the hard stuff." He explained that any problem that could be mathematically described was essentially an easy problem compared to motivational and values alignment issues with employees, where the greatest opportunities and benefits reside. Take a long-term view of aligning all employees toward common goals. Protect the knowledge in the organization through these long-term committed employees.

Employers, particularly in healthcare, have a responsibility to their existing employees as they pursue lean production or any other quality improvement/cost reduction strategy, for example, reengineering, Six Sigma, or TQM. At the beginning of a lean implementation, it's a good idea to announce that no layoffs will result from these efforts. Otherwise, employees will be reticent to cooperate fully with the improvement efforts. The Toyota plant in Fremont, California, has both a no-layoff clause as well as no-strike clause in its union contract to foster continuous improvement and cost reduction. Each healthcare administrator has an ethical responsibility to do everything in his or her power to retain all employees who are functioning at a defined level of good performance. If necessary, a hiring freeze should be implemented early on to retain and, if necessary, redeploy current good employees as opposed to hiring new employees. Attrition or voluntary early retirement may also be used to continually move toward leaner processes. If job changes occur as a result of cost reduction and process improvement, let existing employees know up front that they will have first preference over new hires for any new positions that become available for which they are qualified.

Respect each employee as an important contributor to improvement of quality, cost, and the organization itself. Creating an environment of respect for the employee is the core upon which a successful lean production system is built. Everyone's ideas, suggestions, and opinions are equally important.

Part II

Reduce Healthcare Cost and Improve Quality by Using Toyota Lean Production Methods

3

38 Steps to Improve Cost and Quality in the U.S. Healthcare System

This book will continue by dealing primarily with reducing the cost and improving the quality of healthcare processes. If we improve each of the detailed process steps in how we deliver healthcare, we can thus improve overall healthcare cost and quality. The methods I describe are primarily the same methods used by Toyota Motor Company and other "lean producers." This book won't further pursue the macro system for financing the delivery of healthcare. It also doesn't talk about HMOs, PPOs, Medicare, Medicaid, or other payer systems. Those subjects are highly politically charged on their own. Instead, I will address process improvement methods that may be applied to any healthcare system regardless of payer.[1] I acknowledge that the aging of America and the introduction of new and better technologies are contributing to higher health insurance premiums, but there is little doubt that healthcare processes themselves can be made much more efficient and cost-effective.

I now present 38 steps to improve healthcare cost and quality based on Toyota lean production methods, the advice of lean advocates and quality experts such as W. Edwards Deming, Peter Drucker, Joseph Juran, Philip Crosby, Taiichi Ohno, Shigeo Shingo, Iwao Kobayashi, James Womack, and Don Berwick, and my own 30 years of experience with process improvement in healthcare.

Define value from the perspective of the patient (customer)

Value from the patient's perspective means easy access to appointments, no wait times, timely reports, timely decisions, good outcomes, courtesy, reasonable costs, and so on. A technical definition for a *value-added task* is one that satisfies all of the following:

- It is an activity.

- It is requested by or important to the patient. (In other words, it's something the patient is willing to personally pay for.)

- It changes the thing being processed.

- It is done right the first time. There is no rework or waste.

Use focus groups and surveys to clarify exactly what patients define as value to themselves. Find out what, when, where, and how much the patient actually requires versus what is actually being delivered. Would an uninsured patient choose to pay for a particular process step, activity, or feature? If not, consider eliminating it. Does building a fancy new healthcare facility that looks like the Taj Mahal provide true value to the patient? Does that expensive fountain in the lobby provide true value to the patient, especially one of the 45 million uninsured? Do expanded hospital services provide true value to the patient and community even if similar, high-quality services are already available at a nearby competitor's hospital? How do we properly align the goals of neighboring hospital systems? What is the primary goal of a healthcare provider? Is it to increase its bottom line and market share? Or should the true goal be to cost-effectively and measurably improve the health status of the community? Hospital boards and top executives need to do some soul searching to answer these questions.

It would be wise for key healthcare leaders to meet periodically with their competitors and ask the question, "How can we cooperatively serve the patients in our region more cost-effectively?" They might begin with a jointly funded transport bus to visit most major providers in a region. There could be a shared ambulance and helicopter agreement designed to take the patient to the nearest appropriate healthcare site, as in Seattle, Washington. Or, there might be a common patient ID card with shared insurance and demographic information that is machine readable like a credit card to speed a patient's visit to any provider. They might progress toward noncompeting centers of excellence at each competitor with the competitors literally referring to one another. One competitor might say, "We'll focus on these centers of excellence, and compete less with you as you focus on those." Or, if a piece of new equipment is extremely expensive, "Is there a way to possibly utilize just one for the benefit of all patients in the region?" Based on commitment and cooperation, it is possible for a shared vision for affordable healthcare to become a reality.

 # Map the patient's value stream

A patient's *value stream* is defined as all of the actions, both value-creating and non-value-creating, required to bring the patient from admission through discharge and follow-up. A value stream map is a diagram identifying all the activities needed to receive, care for, discharge, and follow a patient. These include actions to process information for the patient and actions to guide the patient toward a desired outcome. A value stream may be mapped as a flowchart of process steps or as a block diagram showing the relation of all physical locations and objects involved.

The actions within a patient value stream map can be divided into three categories: those that definitely provide patient value, those that provide business value but little or no patient value, and those that provide no value whatsoever. Once the patient's value stream is mapped, the challenge is to provide the patient value-added steps while removing all non-value-added steps and minimizing all business value-added steps. Ask if a patient without health insurance would likely choose to pay for a particular step. If not, try to eliminate it.

Improvement goals include eliminating waiting times, streamlining meetings, minimizing inventories, and minimizing transport wherever possible for all patients, staff, procedures, and supplies. Consider putting a pedometer on a typical patient or staff member, record the transport distance, and then proceed to minimize it. Transport is inherently non-value-added and must be reduced or eliminated wherever possible. (See step 22 for more on eliminating waste.)

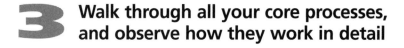

Walk through all your core processes, and observe how they work in detail

Go see your work process for yourself. Understand your work processes thoroughly, even if it means observing for days. Numbers will never substitute for the understanding gained from actually being there. Consider actually performing the job yourself, if possible, to further increase your understanding. Require that supervisors and managers periodically do the actual value-added work, so that they are intimately familiar with all operations and can identify the steps that don't add value.

Personally verify relevant data. Then let everyone think, speak about, and improve processes from personally verified experience and observations. Even high-level managers, vice presidents, and presidents should periodically observe processes in detail, target improvements, and then later verify that the improvements are achieved and maintained.

Seriously consider creating an internal observation team that includes the manager or supervisor of an area along with selected employees and improvement facilitators. Create this observation and improvement team from internal staff as opposed to using expensive external consultants. Focus on removing all waste and creating continuous flow. You will be amazed by what you see if you just take the time to carefully look. (See step 16.)

Implement Toyota-style lean production methods

Establish a continuous flow of work and eliminate delays and waits wherever possible. Clearly state a goal of cutting patient waiting time to zero or at least target a maximum wait-time standard. Post that standard in all areas. A waiting room sign could read, "If you have been waiting more than 20 minutes, please inform the front desk person." With patients flowing more steadily and smoothly through needed treatment areas, the size of waiting rooms and even the treatment areas themselves may be reduced. Continuous flow minimizes patient wait time and treatment time. Likewise, strive to reduce to zero the amount of time any work project is sitting idle. Wherever possible, implement continuous flow for all patients, supplies, materials, process steps, and work projects. Continuous flow will quickly bring process problems to the surface for quick resolution.

It may be important to use a high-quality, coordinated scheduling system to control smooth patient flow throughout the entire organization. Effective patient scheduling is one place where computer technology is well applied. Investing in efficient patient scheduling is likely to be an investment in efficiency. Analyze the situation carefully, however, because a simple pull system that essentially moves the patient through necessary treatment steps in a continuous manner may simplify scheduling without investing in additional technology.

A *pull system* is where the patient (customer) pulls value (toward themselves) from preceding upstream activities. So if the patient needs a major activity performed, that need would automatically pull all required resources and value directly to the patient. Patients should quickly draw all needed services to themselves as they move through their treatment experience. A pull system will provide patients with what they want, when they want it, and in the amount they want.

Recognize that Toyota does not use a complex computerized scheduling system when moving automobiles through the manufacturing process. Instead, the automobiles move smoothly between each process step with all supplies and inventory provided just in time via the use of *kanbans,* which are discussed in step 22 under

"Excess Inventory." So, wherever you can, create a simple pull system to efficiently move patients through their treatments, instead of using a complex or automated scheduling system.

An identifying (kanban) card may be used for patients being treated that will immediately pull services to that patient at each step in their treatment. For example, a receptionist can give a kanban card (with the patient's ID number written on it) to an x-ray patient on first arrival at the reception desk. After an x-ray is complete, the patient returns the card to the receptionist. The card is a signal for the receptionist to immediately notify the doctor to see the patient (since the x-ray is already viewable over the digital x-ray system). This signal for the physician to see the patient is automatic without the need to repeatedly ask additional questions of the patient or staff. This use of a simple kanban card can quickly and easily draw many other services immediately to patients as they move through each of their tests and treatments. Again, this can be done without a costly computerized tracking system.

Please also recognize that patient care paths are designed to pull value to the patient in a scheduled manner. Carefully scrutinize each care path so that its execution becomes nearly automatic.

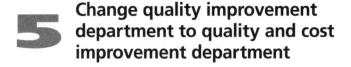 ## Change quality improvement department to quality and cost improvement department

This new quality and cost improvement department will now help stop skyrocketing healthcare costs. Merge the past quality improvement department with any existing industrial or management engineering functions, decision support/data analysis functions, and performance improvement education functions into a single newly named quality and cost improvement department. To help stop skyrocketing healthcare costs, this newly named department will focus equally on improving both cost and quality.

Change the name of the hospital's main quality council that reports to the board of directors to quality and cost improvement council. This quality and cost improvement council will create a vision of continuous improvement for the entire organization and meet at least monthly to solidly and visibly support that vision, create a policy and procedure statement for the improvement process, publish a new quality and cost improvement manual, and suggest objectives for future employee teams. This quality council, in concert with the hospital board, will set objective cost and quality goals at least yearly. A sample goal could be, "There will be no hospital cost increase this year" or, even more commendable, "We will achieve our quality objectives and simultaneously reduce cost per adjusted patient discharge by five percent per year for the next five years." Restructure cost- and quality-related departments and committees as shown in Figure 3.1.

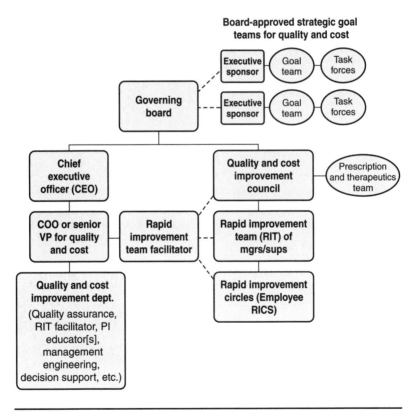

Figure 3.1   Organizational structure for quality and cost improvement.

6 Change the name of the quality improvement manual to quality and cost improvement manual

This manual will not only present quality improvement techniques, but also cost improvement techniques for use throughout the organization.

7 Educate every employee about the basic strategic plan of the organization

It's easy to give each employee a wallet-sized business card that summarizes the organization's current strategic objectives. One side of the card should also be used to record the employee's individual objectives (that are aligned with the organization's objectives). An annual brochure may further clarify the organization's mission, values, and organizational and individual objectives. Each objective should have a what, when, why, how, and by-whom description. In addition, I recommend displaying the organization's mission, values, and strategic objectives for each employee to see in the cafeteria and as they log in to any computer. By having every employee understand the organization's mission, values, and strategic objectives, and how their own objectives align with them, everyone gets moving in the same direction. Visibly and verbally share these items frequently among all employees.

8 Establish an improvement plan with goals to be accomplished by specific people and due dates

Incorporate parts of this improvement plan into your organization's strategic plan. The hospital's main quality and cost improvement council should approve this improvement plan and its objectives and due dates. The hospital board should also receive a copy of this plan for its review and approval. Patient focus groups and survey results would strongly influence the direction of this plan. A Toyota plant has a clear goal that is shared by all, for example, to be first in class in the next J.D. Power survey. Similarly, a hospital may have related Baldrige, ISO 9000, JCAHO, or benchmarking achievement goals. A healthcare provider's plan may focus on improving the following specific areas and core processes. Each core process is labeled patient value-added (PVA) or business value-added (BVA), depending on whether the patient would normally want to pay for it or not.

- Staff scheduling to match patient loads (PVA)

- Productivity monitoring (BVA)

- Core process improvement

  - Admission (BVA)

  - Emergency room treatment (PVA)

  - All patient scheduling processes, for example, inpatient and outpatient (BVA)

  - Outpatient treatment (PVA)

  - Ancillary testing, for example, lab, x-ray (PVA)

  - Surgical treatment (PVA)

  - Medical treatment (PVA)

  - Nursing care process (PVA)

  - Therapy treatments (PVA)

  - Medication process (PVA)

  - Discharge (BVA)

  - Billing (BVA)

- Pharmaceutical cost reduction (PVA)

- Defect reduction, for example, medication errors, infections, falls, medical procedure errors, billing errors (PVA)

- Supplies and materials cost reduction; for example, inventory reduction and improved control (PVA)

- Idealized design of physician office practices (PVA)

- Rapid improvement team goals and initiatives (PVA)

- Patient access to services throughout a region (PVA)

- Strategic initiatives to support quality and cost improvement (PVA)

- Organizational redesign of supervisory and administrative structures (BVA)

- Minimizing financial losses in typically nonprofitable departments (BVA)

- Cost-effective facility design and management (PVA/BVA)

- Information systems redesign to support quality and cost improvement goals (PVA/BVA)

9 Implement a simple scorecard for the entire healthcare organization

Use a simple scorecard to monitor cost and quality improvement in the entire organization and to hold the gains. This scorecard is designed to show how efficiently the healthcare provider is operating in terms of numbers of patients seen, staffing provided, and cost per patient. A simple daily scorecard is shown in Figure 3.2. Strive to keep all your key performance reports to just one or two pages, even for financial indicators. Quality indicators such as medication errors, incidents, defects, and so on, may be added as a second page to the scorecard. This daily scorecard may be a simple spreadsheet that is available online for all to see. It can quickly show where the organization needs to take daily corrective action to improve cost and quality. Graphical monitoring may be added.[2]

Hospital Daily Staffing Report—Week Starting _____	Sun	Mon	Tue	Wed	Thur	Fri	Sat
1. Census							
Med/Surg							
Obstetrics							
ICU							
Nursery							
Total							
2. Visits							
Emergency							
Surgery							
L&D							
Total							
3. Total Nonproductive FTEs							
Med/Surg							
Obstetrics							
ICU							
Nursery							
Emergency							
Surgery							
L&D							
Nursing Admin.							
Total							
4. Total Productive FTEs							
Med/Surg							
Obstetrics							
ICU							

Figure 3.2   A simple daily scorecard.

10 Use a simple scorecard to monitor each department

Use a simple scorecard to periodically (for example, monthly) monitor the level of cost and quality within each department, service, or process to be improved. Figure 3.3 illustrates a scorecard that has the major headings of volume, productivity, quality, and cost. Also, roll up multiple departmental scorecards monthly into a single hospital-wide scorecard. Each department/service can easily maintain this type of scorecard using a spreadsheet program or by using a paper form as shown in Figure 3.3. Each scorecard should contain less than 25 indicators on just one or two pages to keep it simple. You may adapt the departmental scorecard to record measurements monthly, weekly, or daily, depending on the nature of the improvements desired. The scorecard may be posted or displayed where every employee can see it. This supports the Toyota principle of visual control, where all the processes and important parameters of a working department are visible to the workers.

Measurement and inspection are inherently not value-added and are not necessary if the organization, department, service, product, or process works perfectly as designed every time. A patient would generally not want to pay for the effort it takes to monitor a process and might rightly expect the process to be done right the first time and every time. For those things that don't work perfectly every time, however, we need a scorecard to improve them and to then verify that we have improved them. It's key to focus on sustained improvement rather than just measurement. After we are comfortable that the newly improved department, service, product, or process is working consistently in the way we want, we can use the scorecard less frequently (for example, quarterly) to ensure that operations haven't deteriorated. Or we can selectively eliminate certain scorecards or indicators completely if we have full confidence that the improvements are built-in to last.

For department _____								
Indicators	**Target**	**Jul**	**Aug**	**Sep**	**Oct**	**Nov**	**Dec**	**Etc.**
1. Volume								
A. Average daily census								
B. Average daily procedure count								
C. Average daily visits (outpatient)								
2. Productivity								
A. Productive hours care per day								
B. Productive hours care per procedure								
C. FTEs/occupied bed								
3. Quality								
A. Number of defects								
Medication errors								
Infections								
Falls, etc.								
B. Number of incident reports								
C. Lawsuits								
D. $ cost of A + B + C								
E. Patient satisfaction results								
4. Cost								
A. Cost per CMI adjusted discharge								
B. Average cost per patient day								
C. Average cost per procedure								
D. Percent understaffed or overstaffed								
E. Cost of understaffing or overstaffing								
F. Total patient value-added hours								
G. Total hours worked								
H. Ratio of F/G % value-added Total patient value-added								
I. Salary $								
J. Total salary $								
K. Ratio of I/J %								

Figure 3.3 Departmental scorecard.

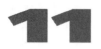

The board of directors initiates selected strategic quality and cost improvement goals

In reality some managers and supervisors may heartily believe they already have a lean staff and may see process improvement projects as a superfluous thing. Some may feel that process improvement is not a high priority compared to their day-to-day management and firefighting activities.

A good way to overcome this reticence is for the organization's board of directors to initiate selected *strategic quality and cost improvement goals* annually. For example, the board may identify and approve six or more strategic quality and cost goals for the year. The board appoints a senior executive to sponsor each of these goals. The board approves specific success measures for each goal; for example, to reduce outpatient waiting time from arrival to lab draw to 10 minutes with results reported to physician within one hour for the patient's visit or to reduce outpatient x-ray waiting time to 10 minutes with results reported to physician within 40 minutes (using digital x-ray). I am aware of a very large clinic that consistently achieves both these quality goals. The senior executive sponsor forms a strategic goal team that meets monthly to review action plans and charter improvement projects (task forces) to achieve the board's objectives. You may call these board-approved "strategic goal teams." The improvement project task forces report monthly to the executive sponsor's strategic goal team, which redirects, approves/ rejects recommendations, and makes resource allocations. The executive sponsor reports back to the board quarterly on progress made by the strategic goal team and its task forces. Any task forces reporting to a strategic goal team are generally short-term do-it groups (DIGS).

It's important to have a sunset date spelled out within the charter of each board-approved strategic goal team. As you might imagine, many projects and task forces may be initiated by the board-approved strategic goal teams. However, it still remains important to actively encourage proposals from frontline rapid improvement teams (RITs) and rapid improvement circles (RICs) that report their results to the hospital's main quality and cost improvement council.

Again it's very important to share all team charters among all the teams to avoid redundancy. To that end, the vice president of quality and cost should be an ad hoc member of the board, to be aware of all board-initiated strategic quality and cost improvement goals and their executive sponsors.

The diagram in Figure 3.1 illustrates the organizational structure for improving quality and cost and includes board-approved strategic goal teams. *It is critical to build such an ongoing quality and cost improvement structure into the entire organization, so that it continually and automatically functions within the organization.*

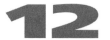 # Create an RIT to make quick cost and quality improvements

Each RIT member is to rapidly achieve and document significant cost and quality improvements at least monthly for a period of approximately one year. An RIT is composed of all department managers and/or supervisors in the organization. All areas are targeted for cost and quality improvement. The team meets on a biweekly or monthly basis. RIT members will later recruit frontline employees into improvement teams.

Give each RIT member a goal of reducing their budget by approximately three percent (to 10 percent) within one year. Or, alternatively, ask each team member to achieve a documented benchmark status of being in the top 25 percent of all comparable departments across the United States in terms of cost and quality. Each team member then documents a specific cost reduction/quality improvement on at least a biweekly or monthly basis until they achieve their goal. That is, each team member actually achieves an improvement every two weeks to a month, not just entertains an idea. They each submit these improvements to the RIT facilitator by completing a cost and quality improvement form. An RIT that I facilitated a few years ago achieved $3.5 million in cost reductions in six months, with a projected three-year savings of $14 million without any layoffs. Comparable success can be achieved by any committed healthcare organization.

A reasonable cost and quality improvement goal would be to achieve best 25th percentile benchmark status or, alternatively, a dollar cost reduction of approximately $4,000 per occupied bed per year. Benchmark values are available from companies such as VHA, Premier, Solucient, or Hewitt Associates. Don't spend excessive time creating and maintaining complex benchmarking systems. They only tell you where you've been. The only way to progress is to take action to improve processes. So, use simple benchmarks like comparing FTE's per adjusted patient day or cost per CMI adjusted discharge. See the simple benchmarking chart for automakers that appears in Appendix A. You can similarly create a simple benchmark comparison among healthcare providers. It's better to spend your time carefully observing and improving processes rather than maintaining complex benchmarking systems.

Form a parallel team to address the rising cost of prescription drugs and other advanced diagnostics and treatments (for example, radiology). This pharmacy and therapeutics team, like the RIT, should report directly to the hospital's main quality and cost improvement council, which will help set specific goals for both.

A study performed by PricewaterhouseCoopers in 2002 found that 22 percent of rising costs in healthcare was due to the increased costs of prescription drugs and other advances in diagnostics and treatment. Yet pharmaceutical companies spend huge sums on advertising campaigns for their products. Pharmaceutical costs are even more troubling since Americans pay, on average, twice the amount for the same common drugs as do the French and Italians. Similarly, Americans pay, on average, 78 percent more than Swedes, 74 percent more than Germans, and 67 percent more than Canadians for the same prescription drugs. This has led to a thriving business in Americans purchasing their prescriptions via Canada. Rising drug costs together with rising hospital costs are the two biggest causes of increasing healthcare costs, both of which must be addressed head on.

The RIT has a senior administrative leader (for example, a vice president or chief operating officer [COO]) who reports directly to the president/CEO. The RIT also has a facilitator/coordinator who understands and can train team members in cost reduction and process and quality improvement techniques. Given adequate knowledge, the senior administrative leader and the RIT facilitator may in fact be the same person. Alternatively, the RIT facilitator may be the head of the hospital's cost and quality improvement department or its designee. The point is that the RIT facilitator should report at a high level in the organization to illustrate the organization's commitment to improvement. The facilitator, all RIT members, plus the complete management team, the board, and all employees must be visibly committed to rapid cost and quality improvement. One can't simply ask employees and physicians to shoulder extra improvement work without first building complete buy-in from the board and all hospital administrators and managers.

The chair of the RIT, who may be the vice president of quality and cost improvement or COO, should be a standing member of the hospital's main quality and cost improvement council that reports to the board. The hospital's main quality and cost improvement council helps set major organizational goals for the RIT. The RIT facilitator may also be a member of the hospital's quality and cost improvement council. (See Figure 3.1.)

The RIT facilitator also provides RIT members with continuing education at team meetings and may elicit the help of consultants having the necessary skills. The facilitator and/or consultant teach team members a problem-solving methodology along with Toyota lean production methods. All vice presidents and the CEO are invited to selected RIT training sessions so they too absorb the new improvement methods. There are many problem-solving methodologies. Table 3.1 presents basic problem-solving methodologies, while Table 3.2 presents improvement philosophies. Toyota lean production is an improvement philosophy or framework that is implemented around a problem-solving methodology. What's most important is not the particular improvement philosophy and problem-solving methodology selected, but rather the simple commitment of the organization to demonstrably pursue continuous cost and quality improvement goals as part of its ongoing mission and values. Still, it is important for the organization to endorse and publish its quality/cost improvement methodology and philosophy, and to eventually train all employees to use it in a relentless manner.

Table 3.1   Basic problem-solving methodologies.

I. Guided design	II. Plan, do, check, act	III. Focus PDCA	IV. Juran	V. Failure mode and effects analysis (FMEA)	VI. Six Sigma using DMAIC
1. Recognize problem.	1. Plan activities to improve a problem or process.	1. Find the process to improve.	1. Identify the problem.	1. Perform a detailed review of the product or process. Team may be used.	1. Define: Establish team and charter; identify sponsor and resources.
2. Define the problem.	2. Do—implement the improvement activities.	2. Organize (a team) to improve the process.	2. Establish the team.	2. Brainstorm all ways it can fail.	2. Measure: Confirm team goal; define current state; collect and display measures/data.
3. Identify alternative solutions.		3. Clarify understanding of the process.	3. Diagnose the cause.	3. List potential effects of each failure mode.	
4. Consider consequences of major alternative solutions.	3. Check to see if the activities really do result in improvement.	4. Understand the root causes of variation in the results of the process.	4. Remedy the cause.	4. Assign 1 to 10 severity rating for each effect. 10 = high.	3. Analyze: Determine process capability and speed; determine sources of variation and time bottlenecks.
5. Choose alternative for implementation, or rank the alternative solutions according to step 4.		5. Select the process improvement.	5. Hold the gains.	5. Assign 1 to 10 probability of occurrence rating for each failure mode. 10 = high probability.	
6. Implement the selected alternative.	4. Act—Either accept the final results or modify the plan in step 1 again and repeat the PDCA cycle.	6. Plan.	6. Replicate solution in other similar settings.	6. Assign 1 to 10 detection rating for each failure mode and/or effect. 10 = not detectable.	4. Improve: Generate ideas; conduct experiments; create straw models; develop action plans; implement.
7. Evaluate and control implementation.		7. Do.	7. Nominate new problems (i.e., return to step 1.)	7. Calculate risk priority number (RPN) for each effect. Severity # × Occurrence # × Detection #.	5. Control: Develop control plan; monitor performance; mistake-proof process.
8. Return to step 1 until desirable/optimal solution is obtained.		8. Check.		8. Prioritize failure modes for action via RPNs.	
		9. Act.		9. Take action to eliminate/reduce the high RPN failure modes.	
Remark: In addition consider:		Repeat PDCA steps 6 through 9 until a final solution is obtained. (PDCA described in prior column.)		10 Calculate the resulting RPNs as the failure modes are reduced or eliminated.	
A. Use team if desirable.					
B. Resources available, as these may mean choosing a solution that may be second best.					
C. Constraints on the situation, as these may also mean choosing a solution that may be second best.					

Table 3.2 Improvement philosophies (that is, framework).

VII. Deming	VIII. Crosby	IX. Baldrige	X. ISO 9000	XI. Lean Toyota Production System
1. What are we doing and why, that is, state mission and values.	1. Management commitment.	1. Leadership.	1. Management responsibility.	1. Respect employees (mutual respect).
2. Improve quality.	2. Quality improvement team.	2. Strategic planning.	2. Quality system principles.	2. Permanent quality/cost improvement structure.
3. Cease dependence on mass inspection.	3. Quality measurement.	3. Customer and market focus.	3. Document control.	3. Cross-trained employee work teams.
4. Don't buy on price alone, but rather on how much you have to pay over the life of the product.	4. Calculate cost of quality.	4. Information and analysis.	4. Purchasing.	4. Improvement plan.
5. Constantly improve every process.	5. Quality awareness.	5. Human resource focus.	5. Identification and traceability.	5. Employee goals with strategic goals.
6. Train employees well using best-practice skills.	6. Corrective action.	6. Process management.	6. Control of processes and production.	6. Quality and cost improvement manual.
7. Show ethical leadership.	7. Zero-defect planning.	7. Business results.	7. Inspection and testing.	7. Continuous flow.
8. Replace fear with trust.	8. Supervisor training.		8. Nonconformance.	8. Visual workplace.
9. Remove barriers among staff areas. Cooperate throughout the organization so that all can win.	9. Zero defects day.		9. Corrective action.	9. Sequence and standardize work.
10. Eliminate slogans, exhortations, and arbitrary targets.	10. Goal setting.		10. Transport.	10. Quick changeovers.
11. Eliminate numerical quotas.	11. Error-cause removed.		11. Quality records.	11. Quality in station.
12. Remove barriers to pride and workmanship.	12. Recognition.		12. Internal audits.	12. Employees stop/fix defective processes.
13. Institute education and self-improvement.	13. Repeat from step 1 through 13.		13. Training.	13. Eliminate all waste: a. Overproduction. b. Poor staff utilization. c. Defects and rework. d. Waits and delays. e. Transportation. f. Unnecessary motion. g. Inventory. h. Overprocessing.
14. Accomplish a transformation to achieve the aim of the business.			14. Follow-up.	14. Help suppliers improve.
			15. Statistical techniques.	15. Hold all gains.
				16. Automate with ROI.

The RIT meets biweekly for about a year or until the members are no longer able to achieve significant cost and quality improvements. After a year, they should have already captured most of the low-hanging fruit in terms of cost and quality improvement opportunities that they can individually see. At some point they need to be reenergized to accomplish more with the help of their frontline employees.

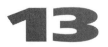

Encourage RIT members to implement Toyota-style work teams

At Toyota, each worker is called a team member since they work all day in small teams of three to eight employees. All team members work near one another and are cross-trained to rotate so as to avoid repetitive stress, add desired variety to their jobs, and so they can cover for and help one another when needed. Creating an effective team is not always easy, as it means that the workers learn a wide variety of skills. In addition to multiple assembly functions, Toyota team members also do housekeeping, minor tool repair, and quality checking, that is, they are multifunctional. Being multifunctional is very efficient in that it eliminates handoffs. Finally, some of the team members periodically have time set aside for suggesting ways to improve processes.

Each team has a team leader, an hourly worker selected by management rather than elected by their coworkers. The team leaders are there to provide team members with whatever they need to do their jobs safely and effectively. A team of three to eight workers and its team leader are referred to as a work team.

There is also a group leader (analogous to a hospital manager or supervisor) who works with a number of teams. A group leader might work with up to eight teams with a grand total of less than 60 employees. The group leader also works alongside the other team leaders and members. Each team leader will immediately help a team member solve a problem. If necessary, the group leader will join in, and if they still can not solve the problem, they will all get together with the hourly and salaried labor reps and work together side by side in the team involvement office to quickly solve the problem. Toyota uses this team work and immediate problem-solving structure every day in its plants and, in particular, in the Freemont, California, plant, which is called New United Motor Manufacturing, Inc. (NUMMI). The NUMMI plant was established in 1984 as a joint venture between Toyota and General Motors Corporation. NUMMI has helped change the U.S. automobile industry by introducing a team-based work environment as well as the Toyota Production System (TPS). The current NUMMI facility was once solely a General Motors facility (GM Fremont) that had been described by one GM manager as the "worst plant in the world." In 1982, GM Fremont closed its doors. Toyota NUMMI began production at the old GM Fremont facility in 1984, with the same union leadership and approximately 85 percent of the workforce comprised of former GM Fremont employees. Within two years, NUMMI was more productive than any other General Motors plant and had quality that rivaled its sister Toyota plant in Japan. If a failed U.S. automaker can remake itself using TPS into a world-class lean producer with highest quality, so too can any hospital, clinic, or health system.

Today, NUMMI is a company with 5500 team members who produce three award-winning vehicles in the United States: Toyota Corolla, Toyota Tacoma, and Pontiac Vibe. In 2002, NUMMI began producing the right-hand drive Toyota Volz, which is exported to Japan. NUMMI has a collaborative partnership with the United Auto Workers and has five core values: teamwork, equity, involvement, mutual trust and respect, and safety. NUMMI was first to demonstrate the success of the Toyota teamwork system in the United States, and other U.S.-based Toyota plants have since followed.

Ask for volunteers among RIT members who wish to try the Toyota teamwork approach in their departments. Certain large hospital departments are particularly amenable to using Toyota-style work teams to better organize daily work. Examples include surgical operating rooms, nursing units, the emergency department, the laboratory, radiology, the pharmacy, physical therapy, medical records, word processing/transcription, food service, and human relations. The advantages of using the Toyota teamwork structure include: fast problem solving, task variety for workers sharing multiple jobs,

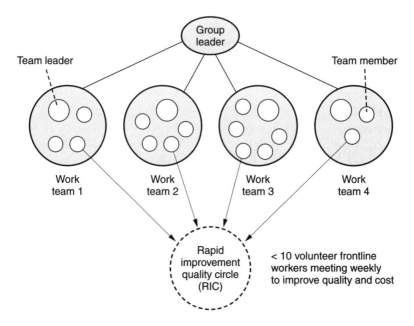

The above structure includes four work teams of three to eight cross-trained workers (team members) with a team leader (larger circle) and group leader (largest oval) and a weekly quality circle (dashed circle) of workers.

Figure 3.4   The Toyota-style work teams of cross-trained employees.

flexibility of cross-trained workers to cover for one another, and built-in ongoing team contributions to continuous quality and cost improvement. The Toyota work team structure is shown in Figure 3.4.

14 Implement rapid improvement circles (RICs) of employees

When the RIT loses energy and creative spirit in approximately a year, then train each RIT member to carry cost reduction and quality improvement down to frontline employees in their respective departments. They may have already begun doing this by volunteering to implement Toyota-style work teams in their departments. Each RIT member is likely to be a department head or supervisor. In addition, train all RIT members to form quality and cost improvement circles in their respective departments anywhere from four to 12 months after the RIT is first formed. These are different than the employee work teams, since they meet only weekly or biweekly. They are synonymous with Toyota's quality circles.

Toyota quality circles are improvement or self-improvement study groups composed of a small number of employees (10 or fewer) and their supervisor. The supervisor's role is likened to that of a coach and enabler, rather than a boss. Quality circles originated in Japan, where they are called *quality control circles.* These quality circles are small groups of volunteer employees who meet on company time to identify, analyze, and solve local problems of their choice and present their solutions to management for implementation approval.

Train RIT members to teach and engage their employees within their new RICs. A current RIT member or their designee chairs each RIC of employees. A key element is that each RIT member teaches their respective RIC members how to do continuous cost and quality improvement and then reports their results back to the RIT. Remember that the RIT is composed of all managers and supervisors of the organization, while each RIC is composed of 10 or fewer frontline employees meeting weekly or biweekly.

After a year, the RIT may meet less frequently, for example, on a quarterly basis. RIT members may have implemented some Toyota-style work teams in their departments to reorganize day-to-day operations. RIT members are now also chairing RICs and are also learning more sophisticated improvement methods at RIT meetings. The RIT helps set goals for the RICs, evaluates their progress, and reports successes and difficulties to the main quality and cost improvement council for the hospital. The weekly or biweekly employee RICs now function as part of the organization's continuous quality and cost improvement effort, while the RIT continues to function as a reporting/training umbrella over the RICs. Employees working day-to-day in Toyota-style work teams also tend to support these efforts since they feed suggestions to the RICs. The RIT or the RICs may also establish task forces designed to quickly solve specific problems within brief periods of time, for example, one to 90 days. For that matter, any of the entities that appear in Figure 3.4 or Figure 3.1 may establish separate task forces reporting to them to solve specific quality and cost problems. Consider the name of "do-it group (DIG)" or go–go group for any short-term task force that is directed at very specific tasks. Each short-term task force would have a written charter containing its goals and sunset date.

As a practical matter, it is wise to manage most improvement task forces via either the RIT, which represents all managers and supervisors in the organization, or RICs, which represent selected volunteer frontline employees. If other committees, teams, or short-term task forces are directed at quality and cost problems within the organization, it is important to have their charters available to all RIT members to avoid duplicating efforts among them.

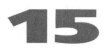

Implement a permanent organizational structure for quality and cost improvement

The structure shown in Figure 3.1 will continuously and permanently carry cost and quality improvement into the future with maximal use of internal staff and minimal expense. This structure is the most important element for the success of ongoing quality improvement and cost reduction. If a hospital can't afford expensive consultants or a large internal quality and cost improvement department with numerous industrial engineers, then existing vice presidents, managers, supervisors, and employees can be trained to do quality and cost improvement within the structure of the internal RIT and its RICs, and board-approved strategic goal teams. All department managers and frontline employees are champions of continuous quality improvement and cost reduction for the entire organization. Newly hired employees are quickly oriented to this continuous quality improvement and cost reduction system so that they can immediately make their contributions toward improvements.

16 Set a goal for each RIC member to produce two to five new suggestions per month

Set a goal for each RIC member (frontline employee) to produce two to five new suggestions each month for cost and quality improvement after their first month or two of participation. Each RIC evaluates its members' suggestions if not overly technical. Otherwise they refer overly technical suggestions to the cost and quality improvement department. In a high-performing RIC, according to Iwao Kobayashi in *20 Keys to Workplace Improvement*, "Group objectives are almost always achieved through the efforts and desires of the members of the group. Everyone is achieving their personal desires while making significant improvement and enjoying each other's association in after-hours recreation."

If an RIC loses energy, allow the RIC members to engage all the employees in their department by also teaching them continuous quality improvement and cost reduction methods. The RIC may also invite new members from other departments so it becomes cross-functional, addressing problems among multiple departments. Cross-functional teams are useful for solving difficult technical problems.

Then extend the goal for every employee in the organization to make two new suggestions for cost or quality improvement each month. Go to employees and ask them what they can do at their workstations to make their jobs easier, and immediately record their suggestions on a suggestion form for them to receive credit. Then do everything you can to make the suggester the implementer. If implementation is beyond their scope, then make them part of the implementation team. Prioritize, and implement the suggestions with the greatest cost benefit. Develop a reward system for employees whose suggestions have been implemented, whether the reward be hours of paid time off, award certificates, meal vouchers, sharing a percentage of the actual savings achieved, or a general gain-sharing program based on achieving annual profit and quality goals for the organization. If you have temporary or traveler employees, also ask for their suggestions and equally reward them. Remember, they may have worked for many other organizations and can share valuable suggestions.

At the Toyota California NUMMI plant, it is interesting to note that in the year 2000, 70 percent of employees participated in turning in approximately 18,000 suggestions, and over 90 percent of them were implemented! In the United States, Toyota employees each contribute about 36 suggestions per year or about three per month. This has achieved millions in savings and employees were rewarded with a payout. They also participated in a gain-sharing program based on company financial goals. Worldwide, the Toyota Corporation in-house suggestion scheme generates over two million ideas a year. Over 95 percent of the workforce contributes suggestions. That works out to over 30 suggestions per worker per year. The most remarkable statistic from Toyota is that over 90 percent of the suggestions are implemented worldwide. In Japan, the average Toyota employee contributes 329 improvement suggestions to the company each year, or more than one per work day.

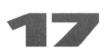

Have a clear award, reward, and recognition program, and communicate negative consequences

As has been mentioned, it's critical to motivate everyone to participate in cost and quality improvement. This means having a clear award/recognition system to recognize outstanding contributions and performance. It means having a reward system to share benefits with those contributing to positive results. This includes award/reward/recognition systems for physicians, practitioners, and other key stakeholders as well as employees. Everyone needs to be involved and motivated.

Develop a gain-sharing program for employees meeting organizational performance goals. This includes frontline employees as well as top administrators. The hospital's board of directors would approve these award/reward/recognition and gain-sharing programs to support its strategic objectives. In addition, publish your positive results in newsletters and newspapers for all to see. Implement a good recognition system to publicly say thank-you to those contributing to your lean successes. Finally, be up front about any negative consequences that may occur if cost and quality improvement targets are missed.

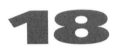

Adopt and teach continuous improvement to as many people as possible in the organization

Permanently embed continuous quality and cost improvement into the organization using Toyota lean production and a problem-solving methodology adopted from Table 3.1. Senior management should learn Toyota-style principles and the improvement methodology first, followed by the RIT members, the RIC members, and then as many employees as possible.

Distribute a short, straightforward, easy-to-understand quality and cost improvement manual for quick reference throughout the organization. The main quality and cost improvement council approves this manual.

Initially use the problem-solving method that best fits your organization's philosophy. It's not so important which problem-solving method you first pick, just that you pick one and begin. Personally, I recommend beginning with the guided design method within the Toyota lean production framework and later migrating to other more complex problem-solving methods from Table 3.1. Guided design emphasizes the thorough consideration of all alternatives, and a slow and deliberate evaluation process followed by a rapid decision and implementation. Invest the time needed with stakeholders to enroll them in the problem-solving process, and obtain their consensus for the chosen solution. Reflect on the shortcomings of previous improvement projects, and avoid those mistakes in the future.

19 The new RIT quickly implements a 5S program

The goal of a 5S program is to organize and clean all workplaces. It's good to have an RIT begin with a 5S clean and organize program as its first initiative. It's quick, about two weeks in length, and demonstrates clearly visible, generally nonthreatening results. It is also a good way to get a quick success for RIT members. Each RIT member can use a simple disposable camera to take before and after 5S pictures to show their dramatic successes. The "after" pictures may be posted on a display board entitled the new Wall of Fame, which was transformed from the "before" Wall of Shame. This can be a fun way to illustrate 5S successes. Alternatively, use a before/after videotape to showcase especially dramatic successes. A 5S program consists of the following steps:

1S. *Sort.* Remove all items from the workplace that aren't needed.

2S. *Set in order.* Arrange items so that they are easy to use, and label them so that they are easy to find and put away. Arrange items to minimize transport time. Use shadow boards or floor outlines to clearly mark the correct locations for storing equipment. A certain area outlined on the floor with a painted stripe to hold a specific amount inventory, supplies, equipment, or work in process will immediately show the naked eye any shortage or excess. To the extent possible, make all available equipment, instruments, and tools visible to the eye as opposed to putting them in closed or locked cabinets. To the extent possible, substitute open shelves and shadow boards for closed cabinets that actually hide things from view.

3S. *Shine.* Clean floors, shelves, counters, and equipment, and keep them clean on a daily basis. Maintain equipment on a frequent, regular basis starting with the most critical equipment first.

4S. Standardize. The first three items are activities, while standardize is the method we use to continue all three of those activities continuously. Document the standard way of how and when we do the first three steps.

5S. Sustain. Make a habit of properly maintaining the standardized methods. If we do the first four steps and come up with a standardized method to keep things orderly, but don't adopt the habit of doing so, all will revert to the way it was before.

A neat, clean, and organized facility has the benefits of higher productivity, produces fewer errors and defects, meets schedules and deadlines better, and is a safer place to work. The following are examples of disadvantages and waste when a 5S program is ignored:

- Excess inventory cost

- Effort to continually rearrange excess inventory

- Unneeded transport of items

- Obsolescence of excess inventory

- Quality defects from aging inventory

- Equipment breakdowns from interfering dirt and debris

- Unneeded equipment and inventory pose a daily obstacle to productive work

- Unneeded items make designing smooth work flow difficult

Appendix C presents a real life healthcare example of 5S as implemented at the VA Pittsburgh Healthcare System. Credit for this example goes to VA Pittsburgh Healthcare System's RN Team Leader Ellesha McCray, CEO Michael Moreland, and Pittsburgh Regional Healthcare Initiative's Communications Director Naida Grunden.

This 5S example may also be found online at the Pittsburgh Regional Healthcare Initiative PRHI Web site http://prhi.org/newsletters.cfm within the December 2003 newsletter. The Pittsburgh Regional Healthcare Initiative at www.prhi.org contains many improvement ideas that may be replicated elsewhere. PRHI is a consortium of institutions and people who provide, purchase, insure, and support healthcare services in the region. Their partners include hundreds of clinicians, 42 hospitals, four major insurers, dozens of large- and small-business healthcare purchasers, corporate and civic leaders, and elected officials. Their goals are:

- Achieving the world's best patient outcomes by

- Creating a superior health system, by

- Identifying and solving problems at the point of care

They are working to achieve perfect patient care in more than a dozen counties in the Pittsburgh area using the following patient-centered goals:

- Zero medication errors

- Zero healthcare-acquired (nosocomial) infections

- Perfect clinical outcomes, as measured by complications, readmissions, infections, and other patient outcomes, in:

  - Coronary artery bypass graft surgery

  - Critical care and emergency medicine

  - Chronic conditions: depression and diabetes

20 Identify unnecessary items using red tags

Implement a red-tag holding area within each department, as well as a final red-tag holding area for the entire organization to temporarily hold excess equipment and inventory that are in question. Make red tags to record item name, date tagged, number of items covered by the tag, reasons why the red tag is attached, department responsible for the red-tagged item, optional value of item, and so on. The best way to carry out red tagging is to do the whole target area quickly; if possible, in one or two days. In fact, many companies choose to complete the entire red-tagging process in one or two days for the entire company. At this stage, just tag the items in question without necessarily evaluating what you are going to do with them. After a limited period of time, for example two weeks, evaluate what you are going to do with each red-tagged item. Options are: keep it in the department or final red-tag holding area for further evaluation, move it to a new location in the work area, store the item away from the work area, or dispose of it (throw away, sell, donate, return to vendor, lend out, distribute to another part of company, or send to a final red-tag holding area). Make a logbook to show the disposition of all red-tagged items. Summarize the results and benefits of the red-tag effort. Often companies that think they need to build more space discover plenty of space by using a red-tag effort.

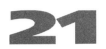

Promote visual control throughout the workplace and organization

Visual control means management by sight, that is, the actual progress of work is always visible. The concept of visual control may be physically extended in the sense of having all departmental work processes as visible as possible to any employee or observer. This means removing as many visual barriers as possible in departments to promote visibly efficient operation. Healthcare organizations generally utilize many managers, supervisors, and administrators, many of whom have private offices. Promoting visual control implies minimizing the number of private offices so that all work activities are visible, and as many employees as possible, including managers and administrators, are visibly doing value-added work that the patient would actually choose to pay for. This implies using more working supervisors and managers who actually share the value-added workload with their employees in addition to managing. Certain private common areas may be reserved for confidential activities such as employee evaluations or rapid problem-solving sessions involving multiple participants. Reducing private office space may be a controversial initiative, but it is consistent with the Toyota principle of visual control.

Visual control also means having inventory, supplies, instruments, and equipment visible to the workers. Closed cabinets, closed supply closets, and opaque enclosures are discouraged. Rather, everything should be visible and within easy reach and access.

Finally, it is also good to have key parameters of work processes visible to the naked eye. A simple control board can show the current work pace and the location of any trouble situations at a glance. Pace is obtained by dividing the total time available per day by the required number to produce per day. So if a medical record area is supposed to process 160 records per 16 hour workday (two shifts), the pace time would be 960 minutes/160 records or six minutes per record. That's the pace needed to accomplish the effort.

Kanban slips attached to supplies show how many are needed, where they came from, and where they are going. Standard worksheets are visible at each work area that show exactly how the process steps are to be performed. A standard worksheet describing process steps will increase efficiency by displaying the workers' best production ideas and also prevents errors and accidents. This is all possible with an inconspicuous standard worksheet. The worksheet will typically contain the cycle time of process steps, the specific work sequence of the steps, and the standard inventory that will be used and produced. *Cycle time* is the time needed to carry out a sequence of steps to produce a given result. *Work sequence* refers to the order of operations that the employee carries out, for example, transporting items, doing activity steps, and removing items or moving them on to the next process. It does not refer to the order of all the processes, just the steps that concern the employee. It is the job of the supervisor to train the workers in the standard procedure. Standard worksheets must be simple, clear, and concise.

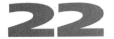 # Eliminate all forms of waste

Recall our earlier estimates that up to 50 percent of healthcare is essentially waste. Taiichi Ohno, father of the Toyota production system, stated, "Eliminating waste must be a business's first objective." The goal is to do only the actions that the patient will actually pay for and to consider everything else as waste. Teach all employees (and RIT and RIC members) to identify waste as "gold, silver, or iron" according to the value of the waste, and then focus on removing or mining the waste that is "gold, then the silver, then the iron." In other words, go after the waste that is most valuable to the organization. In his book *20 Keys to Workplace Improvement,* Iwao Kobayashi says to post a "treasure mountain map" in a central location to show workers where and to what extent waste exists in the workplace. This creates a friendly competition among workers to "mine the mountain of waste." This waste is any activity that adds cost but no customer value to a process. Waste can be categorized as follows.

Overproduction or producing the wrong product entirely

Providing products or services that aren't truly needed wastes resources that could be used to produce products or services that the customer really wants and needs. Verify that the products or services you provide are indeed of the highest value to patients. Recall that according to the *New England Journal of Medicine* study, patients typically receive only 55 percent of recommended care. Is the healthcare provider delivering the appropriate care to the patient in a cost-effective manner?

I usually ask what the charge is for a medical procedure beforehand even though I have insurance. I'm told by my friends that I'm rare in doing so. I'm usually surprised that the physician has only a vague idea of the charge to the patient. I have been surprised by responses like, "I'm a doctor, you'll have to ask the business office."

Physicians and nursing staff being oblivious to actual charges is a disservice to patients. It is wise to post the charges for common procedures and supplies for all physicians and nursing staff to see in their work areas. You'll probably get an "I had no idea" reaction from them. With these patient charges visible to them every day, they will probably begin to utilize those services more cost-effectively. They'll also be able to communicate costs better to patients, especially the uninsured.

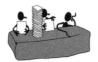

Waste of Overproduction

Producing more and/or faster than needed or producing the wrong product/service

Symptoms	Actual Examples
• Not following care paths	• Patients typically receive 55% of recommended care (NEJM study)
• Performing services patient doesn't need, for example, lab work	• 25% of surgical supplies picked and returned to shelf
• Unbalanced staff scheduling	• Picking OR instruments but not using them so they must be resterilized
• Having more than needed of anything, for example, beds	• Not notifying food service of diet changes and discharges
• Extra floor space utilized	
• Unbalanced material flow	• Repeatedly printing "face sheets" on nursing units
• Backups between departments	

Incorrect utilization of staff

This form of waste has two variations: (a) using the wrong level of staff for a certain task, and (b) under- or overstaffing across the organization. I classify understaffing as a form of waste, as it will lead to burnout and loss of the employee. The wasted costs of rehiring and retraining then follow. Approximately 60 percent of total hospital costs are labor costs. In order to control healthcare costs, it's critical to control labor costs. This means having a responsive staffing system that accurately allocates staff to each work area based on numbers of patients (or procedures) and their acuity, that is, based upon workload. If the workload in an area is excessive at any given time, it's critical to quickly move similarly qualified staff from less utilized areas. Be responsive to shift-to-shift changes in workload. If the workload spikes up, then add staff, but if it dips down, remove staff.

A pool of float staff can facilitate these moves. If workload falls, you may schedule some staff to work on improvement teams and projects. Avoid fixed staffing levels that are not responsive to changing workload. To the extent possible, level out the workload by scheduling patients in a predictable manner, in accordance with the staff that are scheduled. If the patient scheduling system and the staffing scheduling system don't correspond to one another on a day-to-day and shift-to-shift basis, frequent problems will arise.

In order to be most cost-efficient, it is critical that activities be performed by the lowest level of staff (that is, most frontline and lowest paid) who are qualified and skilled to perform the job. In addition, it's very important for any operational decisions to be made at the lowest possible level that is appropriate. Too often, operational changes that can produce immediate benefit are unnecessarily postponed for approval by some executive. It is often a waste of the executive's time, when the decision to implement an improvement could have been made at the level of the work team. It's sufficient for the work team to keep their group leader or manager apprised of improvements being made and to consult with them on controversial changes. This speeds improvement and flattens the organization structure at the same time.

A good example of unnecessary waste is having numerous RNs doing certain operating room tasks that could be performed just as well by techs. Another specific example I observed was an RN who was employed full time exclusively doing repetitive phlebotomy (blood draws). A well-trained phlebotomist would have done the job just as well and more cost-effectively. Cross-training staff, however, to perform multiple tasks is a good way to increase their value and versatility to help out whenever and wherever needed. The simple principles of cross-training staff to be more versatile and having the lowest level of qualified staff performing, managing, and improving tasks are not as rigorously practiced in healthcare as in Toyota lean production. How often do supervisors and mangers assist with frontline healthcare activities?

How often do frontline healthcare staff rotate jobs with team members? At Toyota, a lead worker may lead a continuous improvement team but will also fill in for absent employees or whenever needed to solve immediate production problems. If healthcare workloads are too light, and staff can't easily be moved to areas of greater need, then it's important to immediately offer them the option of time off without pay. The bottom line is that it's critical to achieve balanced and equitable staffing levels throughout a healthcare organization based on the workload present each shift and each day. A system to schedule, allocate, and redistribute staff based on continually changing workload remains a critical element for controlling healthcare costs. A computerized system to schedule and allocate staff may be a good investment to reduce healthcare costs. Or try to develop a simpler nonautomated system to continuously and fairly allocate staff.

Gradually minimize job classifications among employees. This is an emotionally charged issue, but at least try to slowly move toward fewer job classifications. Excessive job classifications and specialization increase idle time, handoffs, and so on. Consolidation of job classifications increases flexibility and thereby reduces those forms of waste. Interestingly, there are just three job classifications at the NUMMI Toyota plant to set team members apart: production, tool and die, and general maintenance worker. This compares to dozens of job classifications at most other U.S. automakers. Team members routinely rotate through different jobs within their small teams. Multifunctional workers eliminate handoffs.

Defects and rework

Defect examples include medication errors, incorrect surgeries, and poor clinical outcomes. Rework examples include retesting, rescheduling, resubmitting lost or rejected insurance claims, rewriting of patient demographics, and multiple bed transfers. All represent unnecessary effort and wasted resources, and contribute to ongoing quality problems. Any type of inspection well after an original process may also be considered rework. All checking is waste and may be prevented by error-proofing the original process. Create a culture to fix the cause of problems immediately as they are encountered. Build a visual system to quickly show when problems arise so they can be immediately fixed. Avoid using a computer screen if it pulls the employee away from doing value-added work. Allow any employee to stop the process and immediately fix a problem. Future occurrences are then minimized. This is what happens in a Toyota plant, with simple *andon* lights signaling the problem on the stopped assembly line. (Andon is the Japanese word for paper lantern.) An andon board (as shown in Figure 3.5) lets supervisors know the location of the problem with a blinking light and a distinct musical tone.

Any employee can stop the line to resolve a problem. "Processes producing 'just in time' do not need extra inventory. So, if a prior process step generates defective parts, the next process step must stop the line. This makes defects immediately apparent. Furthermore, everyone sees when this happens and the defective part is returned to the earlier process. It is an embarrassing situation meant to help prevent the recurrence of such defects," explains Taiichi Ohno in *The Toyota Production System.*[3] Toyota uses a green andon light to show that all is normal, yellow to show when a worker is adjusting something, and red to show if a worker has stopped the line to rectify a problem.

A new production line may stop frequently as problems are resolved, but then begin to run smoothly, continuously, and efficiently. Ultimately, the number of errors will fall, and the line will almost never stop. Today in Toyota plants where every worker can stop the line, it almost never stops and yields approach 100 percent.

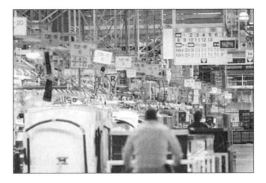
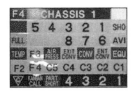

Figure 3.5   This *lighted board* (upper right) shows where an andon cord has been pulled to signal a problem on the line at Toyota Motor Corp.'s plant in Georgetown, Kentucky. If the issue is not fixed before the car reaches the next stage of assembly, the line stops.

Source: Photo and caption reproduced with permission of *The Detroit News.*

Toyota encourages employees to pull the cord, despite the line stoppages, to expose problems and address them quickly. In Toyota's Georgetown, Kentucky, plant, workers pull the line-stop cords 2500 times a shift to signal problems, but actual stoppages only amount to six to eight minutes per shift.[4] Yasuhiro Monden, author of a manual used at Toyota's California NUMMI plant, writes of the assembly line, "It is not a conveyor that operates men; it is men that operate a conveyor."

One may not see lighted boards flashing problems near the ceilings in hospitals or clinics, but in healthcare it's easy for any employee to similarly stop a defective process with a simple explanation to their other team members and a page or phone call to their supervisor, team leader, or manager. At that time they can all ask *why* five times to determine the true root cause of the problem and correct it so that it will never happen again. Unfortunately, this mentality of immediately identifying a problem and permanently eliminating it isn't common enough in health care. Even though Toyota-style andon boards aren't often seen in hospitals, they could be considered in high-production areas like operating rooms, supply processing departments, emergency departments, and nursing units.

Quickly fixing problems as they occur involves having a support system that can quickly put solutions in place. The idea is to resolve the problem as soon as it crops up. Toyota employees all work in small teams of three to eight members who are generally referred to as team members. Each team has a team leader that is selected rather than elected. The team leader is there to provide team members with whatever they need to do their jobs safely and effectively. The team leader does the same work as the other team members, but also coordinates the team and, in particular, fills in for any absent workers, an uncommon concept in U.S. mass production. There is also a group leader over a number of teams, who also works alongside the other team leaders and members.

When someone pulls the andon cord to signal a problem, the team leader may immediately help solve the problem. It is not uncommon to also see maintenance workers picking up production tasks to help with the problem. If necessary, the group leader will join in, and if they still can not solve the problem they will get together with the hourly and salaried labor reps to all work together in the team involvement office to solve the problem.

Taiichi Ohno stated that we should have a system in place that immediately responds to a problem when it occurs. This is a marked contrast to historical U.S. mass production where the assembly line was virtually never stopped, and problems were fixed after automobiles rolled off the end of the line or, even worse, after the customer took possession. At the Toyota NUMMI plant, team members are also each given a personal touch fund of $15 so that they can meet off-hours to further solve problems. Pizza anyone?

Now, many U.S. manufacturing companies are embracing lean to reduce costs even though it may involve wrenching changes. This is a necessity to respond to worldwide competition from low-cost countries such as China and Mexico. These companies are now pushing to have healthcare providers adopt similar approaches to reduce skyrocketing healthcare costs, which are a major expense for them.[5] To avoid conflicts in adopting these approaches within healthcare, it's important to be sensitive to perceived differences in the culture of caring healthcare compared to the culture of manufacturing efficiency. It may take years to fully successfully transfer Toyota lean production methods to certain areas of healthcare, but targeting to begin to do so in months rather than years is advised. There will be starts, stumbles, stops, and even back steps along the way, but improving processes is the key to improving healthcare quality and costs.

Wherever possible, Toyota uses machines that stop themselves if defects are detected (*jidoka* or autonomation). It also requires workers to stop the line if they detect any defect or abnormal condition. The jidoka (quality in station) philosophy shows faith in the team member as a thinker and allows all team members the right to stop the line on which they are working. Jidoka prevents defects from continuing and allows the situation to be immediately investigated and corrected. The idea is to build in quality by preventing any defect from going to the next process. Each worker is an inspector for his or her own work and that of coworkers. This results in a working system that is designed to provide highest quality and lowest cost with minimal inspection.

It is important to mistake-proof (poka-yoke) processes wherever possible. Poka-yoke essentially makes it impossible for a particular defect to occur. Literally translated, the Japanese word *yokeru* means to avoid while *poka* means unintentional error. So *poka-yoke* is translated as avoiding unintentional errors. An everyday life example is a buzzer going off in your car if you open the door with your headlights on. This is a detection poka-yoke that alerts the operator of an error to prevent a defect (the battery going dead). A common prevention poka-yoke is having the unleaded gas tank insert smaller so that the larger leaded pump nozzle can't fit into it. This prevents the error from ever occurring. Think about it. Every time you put gas in your car, you are automatically inspecting that you are using unleaded gas based on the size of the unleaded gas pump nozzle. Another prevention poka-yoke is not allowing a car to start unless the shifter is in the park position.

A healthcare poka-yoke may mean not storing lethal or harmful doses of drugs anywhere, particularly on nursing units, to prevent an overdose. It may mean having equipment that can only be connected in the recommended manner, since the parts will not fit together in any other way, thus avoiding potential injury. It may mean having buzzers on equipment to signal dangerous conditions. It may mean automatically isolating certain infected patients in a manner to prevent further spread of the infection. It may also mean always using disposables to prevent the spread of infection.

Perform root cause analyses to eliminate the causes of defects and rework and implement countermeasures. Like Toyota, ask *why* five times to get at the real cause of the problem. Analyze and/or try different alternatives until the problem is resolved. Maintain a continuous improvement program to minimize defects/rework. Continuously reduce defects to zero.

As shown in Table 3.1, Six Sigma is a quality improvement methodology that follows the DMAIC steps of define, measure, analyze, improve, and control, and its goal is to reduce process variation and eliminate defects. Fortune 500 companies like GE, Motorola, and McKesson implement Six Sigma programs to reduce defect rates to less than 3.4 per million. Six Sigma improvements are driven by data. Six Sigma focuses on projects that will produce measurable business results. Using Six Sigma, GE Capital saved two billion dollars in 1999.

There is nothing magical about Six Sigma, and it shares much in common with other past improvement methods. The *define* step presents a clear explanation of the problem/project. The *measure* step illustrates how much variation there is in the process. The *analyze* step looks at alternatives to improve the process and reduce variation and defects to six sigma targets. The *improve* step implements those changes. Finally, the *control* step ensures that the newly improved processes will not revert to prior excess variability and defect levels. Six Sigma is based upon improving processes by understanding and controlling variation, thus improving the predictability of results. So, study the variation in processes and their defect rates, and systematically minimize both.

Waste of Correction

Inspect and/or repair a defective service or product

Symptoms	**Actual Examples**
• Adverse drug events	• Utilization review, infection control, legal, and risk management inspections
• High infection rates and falls	
• High incidence of bill rejects	• Lack of standardized script at registration
• Frequent rescheduling of office appointments	
• Multiple quality control checks	• Replacing "lost" gowns in OR/nursing
• Patient returns (OR, readmit)	• Inappropriate communication of patient transfer mode with order entry
• Missed shipment/deliveries	
	• Pharmacy refilling "multiple dose" medications

Waits and delays

Organize work so that there are as few delays as possible. Examples of common delays include: waiting for medical appointments, medical assessments, ancillary tests to be performed, test results, bed assignments, surgical and nonsurgical scheduling, presurgical testing, OR prep, payment cycle times, and so on. Unnecessarily monitoring patients or watching equipment operate is another example of waste. When possible, do intermediate steps in parallel at the same time. Study each step and subprocess and reduce its length of time.

Waste of Waiting

Idle time created when people wait for machines, people wait for people, or machines wait for people

Symptoms	Actual Examples
• Unbalanced scheduling/workload	• Waiting on test results
• Idle people or machines	• Surgeons waiting on OR preference card change
• Large waiting rooms	• Outpatient lab draw takes 1.5 hours
• Access to care problems	
• Reduced productivity	• Patients wait between multiple appointments
	• Patients wait for discharge placement

Transportation

The act of moving materials or information around clearly doesn't add any value to the customer or patient. Actually, any transport process in itself is non-value-added and needs to be eliminated or at least minimized.

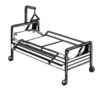

Waste of Transport of Material and Information

Any material or information movement

Symptoms	Actual Examples
• Inappropriate bed assignments on admission	• Temporary warehouses and multiple storage locations
• Having multiple information systems	• Walking intermittent samples to lab or going to get prescriptions
• Excessive medical records pickups and deliveries	• Staff copies patient chart for transfer between facilities
• Extra handoffs of anything	• Finished patient chart walked to financial counselor
	• Multiple copies of surgery schedule distributed daily
	• Every outpatient visit requires driver's license

Unnecessary motion

People and equipment are rarely where they are needed. Searching for things and restacking inventory are examples of the waste of unnecessary motion. Employees stretching and walking to reach materials represents non-value-added activities and waste. Equipment may be difficult to prepare, load, and clean. Regardless of how often a worker moves, it does not mean they have completed meaningful work. An employee may keep busy for hours just looking for things and never accomplish any meaningful work. They are just adding to cost and lengthening service time. All needed supplies and equipment should be nearby the worker. Accomplishing meaningful work means that the worker has completed value-added steps efficiently and with as little motion as possible. Use 5S to standardize, minimize, and organize work environments.

Waste of Unnecessary Motion

Any movement of people or equipment

Symptoms	Actual Examples
• Excess patient transfer/movement	• Searching for anything, for example, equipment
• Convoluted facility and workplace layouts	• Emergency department triage, registration, treatment room, x-ray, financial counselor
• Prolonged pre-op testing times	
• Inconsistent work methods	• Poor workplace layout for patient services
• Reduced productivity	
• Long reach/walk distances	• Locations of fax/copy machines
• Long lead times for anything	

Excess inventory

Minimize the amount of preprocess inventory, in-process inventory, and end-of-process inventory. Set a goal to reduce the total of all inventory in the organization by 50 percent or more. Do not purchase supplies in large lots. Inventory, storage, and handling savings will more than offset savings achieved through volume discounts. Use two containers to hold supplies and inventory at the point of use. When one is emptied, simply send it back to be refilled. The second full container is still there as your safety supply. Size the containers so there are no inventory stock-outs. This system, a *kanban* system, is simple, requires no costly automation, and minimizes the inventory at each site of use. It was invented by Taiichi Ohno of Toyota in the 1950s. "He dictated that parts would only be produced at each previous step to satisfy the immediate demand of the next manufacturing step. As each container carrying parts was used up at a manufacturing step, it was sent back to the previous step, and this became the automatic signal for more parts."[6] This simple idea is enormously powerful, and it eliminates nearly all excess in-process inventories. Alternatively, use a kanban ordering card to pull just the right amount of inventory to the next process step at the time it is truly needed. Kanban cards signal the need for more inventory at the right time and place. This can all be done without complex computer systems.

Minimize all inventories, but maintain safe levels. Savings generated by reducing inventories and supplies will fall directly to the bottom line and immediately increase profits. Imagine the entire organization moving supplies on a series of intersecting, continuously moving conveyor belts. Each conveyor feeds supplies to each work process at the rate of supply consumption for that process and no more. Only when supplies are depleted to minimum safety levels are those supplies replenished in minimum order quantities. Replenishment is initiated only by actual consumption. Try to achieve process steps that require no inventory. After improvement, have employees eliminate any exposed inventory. Many areas in hospitals can take advantage of kanban systems to minimize inventory, including central stores, supply processing department (SPD), pharmacy, food service, nursing units, ORs—virtually any area with inventory. Start with the areas that contain the greatest dollar value of inventories.

A hospital materials manager once boasted to me that he was achieving "26 inventory turns a year." That means that at any given time, the hospital had about two weeks of inventory on hand. In comparison, Toyota typically has an inventory of two hours of parts on hand, which equates to roughly 2500 inventory turns a year. Consider the difference! In his book *The Machine That Changed the*

World, author James Womack presents a chart that shows Toyota having two hours of parts inventory on hand versus two weeks at a General Motors plant in 1986.[7] General Motors, like the hospital materials manager, might also have inappropriately boasted at that time about their inventory efficiency. Yet, Toyota was 100 times more efficient at minimizing its inventory.

I am aware of hospitals that achieve as little as two inventory turns a year. That means they may keep as much as six months of supplies in inventory. Some hospitals consider six turns a year acceptable, which equates to two months of inventory. Retaining this much inventory on hand simply increases cost. Many hospitals try to achieve a national target of 12 to 15 turns a year, while some consider 26 turns a great achievement. Every hospital should continuously strive to reduce inventories to safe but minimum levels.

Another example of Toyota's use of lean inventories is illustrated by the West Coast dock strike of September 2002. At that time I saw a Toyota plant manager from NUMMI on CNN national news. The plant manager commented that his plant only had a day or two of Toyota engines and transmissions on hand even though these were shipped from Japan! Why is it that a Toyota assembly plant in California can operate with only a day or two of critical engines and transmissions from Japan, while a hospital in the United States needs two weeks or more of inventory principally made in the United States?

It is now a challenge for hospital materials managers to safely minimize inventories and have those savings go directly to the hospital's bottom line. A goal of reducing hospital inventories by one-half by using kanban systems is reasonable, as demonstrated by Toyota and other lean producers. Note also that a kanban system is primarily a simple manual system without the need for staff to enter supply orders into sophisticated computer systems.

Use a kanban system to eliminate all the cost and overhead associated with expensive, computerized order entry systems. The kanban is usually a piece of paper in a rectangular vinyl envelope that is divided into three categories:

- Pickup information

- Transfer information

- Production information

This information may also appear on the corresponding container. At a glance, a kanban may also provide: production quantity, time, method, sequence or transfer quantity, transfer time, destination, storage point, transfer equipment, container, and so on.

The first rule of kanban is that the later process goes to the earlier process to pick up items. This reverses the conventional flow of production, transfer, and delivery. The later process must instead take what it requires from the earlier process when it is needed. This sets the pace for the earlier process.

In addition to reducing in-process inventory with kanbans, it's important to reduce the amount of preprocess inventory. I'm aware of one large nonprofit system of 14 hospitals that has reduced the number of items in its inventory catalog from 250,000 to about 70,000 through standardization and value analysis of supplies and equipment. It has reduced its catalog by over 70 percent, and certainly has achieved great savings in the process. It is targeting to have a final catalog of about 35,000 items for its entire health system, which amounts to an 85 percent reduction. That was a target suggested to it by DeLoitte and Touche consultants.

When undertaking such preprocess inventory reduction, it's very wise to create a systemwide value analysis team with membership from all facilities. This systemwide value analysis team would have a similar goal of reducing preprocess inventory by 80 percent and in-process inventory by 50 percent. Remember that these savings will fall immediately to the bottom line and essentially represent profit on the income statement.

Excess inventory just hides a multitude of underlying problems. Kiyoshi Suzaki states, "excess inventory is the root of all evil."[8] To reduce inventory and eliminate these examples of waste, hospital staff must simultaneously expose and correct the underlying problems such as:

- Poor scheduling

- Communication problems

- Production imbalance between departments

- Long setup times

- Long transportation

- Vendor deliveries
- Equipment/instrument breakdown
- Quality problems
- Absenteeism
- Lack of housekeeping and organization

Waste of Inventory

Any supply in excess of just-in-time customer requirements for goods or services

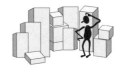

Symptoms	Actual Examples
• Multiple forms, multiple copies, multiple weeks' supplies	• Duplication of supplies in temporary storage areas, patient rooms, closets, and so on
• No standardization of supplies	
• Unused appointment slots	• ED filled entire dumpster from one outdated storage area
• Empty beds	• One surgical services cart alone had $250K of sutures
• Complex tracking systems	
• Multiple storage and handling	• Excessive duplication in OR, SPD, pharmacy, nursing units
• Extra rework/hidden problems	

Excess processing

Unneeded steps are often used to achieve a result. Overprocessing represents waste. Complex registration processes are common examples of excess processing in healthcare. I have seen returning laboratory outpatients go through a very time-consuming, full hospital registration process before having their blood drawn at one hospital, while outpatients at another hospital just provide their name, date of birth, home address, and insurance carrier.

Another example of excess processing is multiple registrations where the patient is asked repeatedly for the same information. Excessive paperwork and entering duplicate information on computer screens are other examples. If a person records information once, there is no need to record it again if systems and forms are well designed. Toyota also tries to build a kind of human intelligence into their machines. If a worker starts a task on one of these machines, they do not have to idly watch the machine do its job. They can go on to another productive task. There are probably examples of staff in healthcare watching a machine, task, process, or patient when careful design could eliminate the need for watching (which is continuous inspection). Designs to remove continuous inspection have to be implemented very carefully so as to improve quality rather than degrade it. These designs may be most successful with equipment; in other words, try to obtain equipment that works so well that there is no need to watch it. Such equipment will immediately and appropriately signal you if there is a problem.

Many types of meetings are also good examples of waste. For example, calculate the expense of a given meeting in terms of the total staff, their hourly salaries, the total time consumed, and their travel time. Always ask the question ahead of time, "What are the goals of the meeting?" and afterward ask if they were accomplished expeditiously. Always have a written agenda stating the meeting goals and agenda items with times and responsibilities allotted for each. Distribute the agenda at least two days ahead of time. The purpose of the agenda is to let members know exactly why they are coming and what will be expected of them at the meeting. Use a simple one-page form to record meeting minutes and results that can be distributed within a day after the meeting. Always ask the question, "Is this meeting something the patient would pay for or does most of it represent a kind of overprocessing waste that a patient would not wish to pay for?"

Similarly, multiple committees within an organization may have overlapping responsibilities. For every committee and task force, it's important to have a written charter defining goals and responsibilities. See the example charter in Figure 3.6. The charter for a task force should include a sunset date after which the task force will no longer meet. A task force is generally considered to be a short-term work group to accomplish specific tasks within a limited time of, say, a few days to 90 days. Standing committees may be a permanent part of the organization with no sunset date. Other nonstanding committees may have multiple goals and a sunset date for accomplishing those goals. Task forces may report to committees. It is important to streamline the overall committee structure to eliminate overlap wherever possible and to choose the membership carefully to appropriately utilize all members. Any underutilized member can be an ad hoc member to be included only when necessary.

Specific challenge (purpose):

Team leader/facilitator:

Executive sponsors:

Core team members:

Recorder:

Primary customer:

Tentative meeting schedule:

Sunset date:

Objectives and goals:

Key questions to answer:

Key activities:

Flowcharts to compose:

Figure 3.6 Sample team charter.

Waste of Excess Processing

Effort that adds no value to the product or service from the customer's perspective

Symptoms	Actual Examples
• Asking the patient the same questions multiple times	• Duplicating physical assessment at triage and in treatment area
• Multiple signature requirements	• Placing OR scheduling information in multiple systems
• Extra copies of forms	
• Duplicate information system entries	• Punching holes in paper to place in patient chart
• Manual distribution of numerous report copies	• Idly watching equipment operate
• Long lead time	
• Reduced productivity	
• Sorting, testing, and inspection	

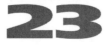 # Reduce specific examples of potential waste

There is much potential for the elimination of waste in healthcare. As a preface to this step, we should all remember that a patient's healthcare is primarily delivered by a physician and nurse(s) and supporting ancillary departments like the lab, the pharmacy, x-ray, and surgery, that provide the needed tests, drugs, therapies, and interventions. There are some other staff categories and some activities that would not exist or would at least be minimized in an ideally designed, highest-quality, lean hospital/clinic.

If a lean healthcare provider delivered best quality, many of the activities and positions discussed below would be less needed. The list is likely only a fraction of what might decrease in a truly lean, highest-quality healthcare organization. Remember Don Berwick's estimate that 40 percent of healthcare is waste, and Jim Womack's estimate that a truly lean organization can reduce labor, space, and inventory by half. It is a challenge for each healthcare provider and each of the following departments to embark on a lean journey of continuous cost and quality improvement to reduce the need for their own services. Just as it is said that a good consultant's job is to make his or her services no longer needed, so too it should be the goal in each of these and possibly other departments to reduce the need for their services by instead improving quality. Still, the organization's principle of respect for the employee would ensure that each good-performing employee would still have a job for which they are qualified. Each of these employees is most likely a good, highly skilled, dedicated worker whose services may be redeployed elsewhere. Here are some examples of activities and positions that may be reduced if the highest quality were built into lean healthcare processes.

Excessive layers of administrators, managers, and inspectors

Scrutinize the numbers of administrators, managers, supervisors, and inspectors. As a challenge, ask your human resources (HR) department to count the number of direct patient value-added employees, the ones who directly service patients and for whom patients are totally willing to pay. HR may use a patient focus group if there are any doubts about a function being patient value-added. In 2000, a hospital HR consulting firm suggested an average target ratio of 16 employees per manager or supervisor when computed across the entire organization. Obviously some departments have many more employees per manager while others have fewer, but organization-wide they suggested the ratio of 16 to one. It would be good to obtain a new benchmark of this ratio in healthcare at this time. For contrast, I recall that Jack Welch targeted an average ratio of 25 to 30 employees per supervisor during his tenure at General Electric.

Then, compute the ratio of direct patient value-added employees divided by total employees. You may find this percentage astounding. In addition, ask HR to compute total salary dollars for the direct patient value-added employees. Then divide that by the total salary dollars for all employees. You may be even more astounded by that percentage. It is an ongoing challenge to continually increase those two percentages.

Utilization review staff and discharge planners

This may be a big example of waste due to inspection. If proper utilization and discharge planning were built into existing patient care processes, then most utilization review positions would go away. Basically, utilization review staffs continually recheck what physicians and nurses are doing so that the patient leaves the hospital in a timely manner so that Medicare/Medicaid reimbursement will be sufficient. Insurance companies may also require utilization review staff to minimize length of stay to match reimbursement. One large hospital where I once worked had about 40 such utilization review staff, most of whom were nurses who could have been potentially providing direct care to patients.

Patient advocate(s)

A patient advocate is a hospital employee who receives patient complaints and then tries to satisfy the angry patient or passes the complaint on to someone who will hopefully prevent a recurrence. In an ideal healthcare delivery system, there would be little need for patient advocates as complaints would be minimal to nonexistent.

The patient advocate position is symbolic of rework in a patient process gone wrong.

Infection control nurses and staff

If ideal sterile techniques were followed, there would be few infections and little need for these infection surveillance staff. A large hospital may have approximately five such staff in a department. These staff monitor and report infections and help educate patient care providers on how to best prevent infections. Not only is there cost associated with these surveillance staff, but there is a far greater cost associated with the consequences of infections to patients. These consequential costs stem from extended lengths of patient stay, the use of specialized drugs, possible isolation, and follow-up interventions. One system of hospitals with a total of 885 beds estimated the consequential costs of infections at over a million dollars per year, not counting the cost of the infection surveillance staff themselves. In a truly lean, highest-quality hospital, this staff would be completely focused on education to avoid all future infections. In the January 4, 2004 *Boston Globe Magazine,* Don Berwick states during an interview that if hospitals would impose a zero-tolerance policy for workers failing to wash their hands, that simple step could save upward of 10,000 lives a year.[9] During my extended career in healthcare, on several occasions I have seen physicians use the men's room and not wash their hands before beginning rounds. True. Use the Toyota principle of immediately responding to every infection (that is, defect) as it occurs to prevent all similar recurrences in the future. Quickly and permanently eliminate identified root causes of infections and then focus infection control staff on continued educational efforts to hold the gains.

Managers, supervisors, and coordinators

If managers, supervisors, and coordinators don't provide direct patient care, are patients usually willing to pay for their services? If care processes were better designed could these non–care providing positions be reduced? Could they be converted to instead provide direct patient care?

Medicare compliance officer and staff

This position is an on-staff inspector to ensure that Medicare regulations are being met. Because of past oversights, it is now a federal requirement to have a Medicare compliance officer. If Medicare regulations were continuously met in a high-quality/high-trust organization, these positions would not be necessary. They have only come into vogue within the last five years.

Legal counsel(s) for patient lawsuits

If highest-quality care and outstanding customer service were consistently provided, there wouldn't be any patient lawsuits and little need for these supporting attorneys.

Safety/risk managers and staff

Again, like lawyers, staff in this department are there to respond to major problems that may lead to patient litigation for the hospital. If quality were built in, there would be no need for this function.

Marketing

Individual healthcare providers may spend hundreds of thousands of dollars annually marketing themselves via mailings, TV ads, and so on. Is this something patients and their employers would willingly choose to pay for? Why is so much advertising needed in healthcare? If we had a national system to equitably distribute healthcare resources, then healthcare providers would not need to use advertising to compete for patients.

Numerous financial analysts/auditors

These analysts essentially watch over all the department managers and how they budget and expend funds. One large, three-hospital system with which I'm familiar had 22 such financial analysts. Why so many inspectors? If good financial management were built into departments, that number could be significantly reduced.

Excess secretaries

Generally, the CEO and each vice president have their own private secretary, and most department heads also have private secretaries. Why so many? A much smaller pool of secretaries that is shared by all would be much more efficient, for example, located within a centralized transcription service and secretarial pool. Or, having one secretary shared among approximately three or more vice presidents or department heads would be much more efficient. Healthcare providers have spent large sums in the past 20 years on personal computers, networks, and software to make communications and secretarial work easier. So, isn't it reasonable to share each secretary among three or more administrators and department heads? Remember that each department head now also has a personal computer to help manage their information and schedules.

Excess information technology

Many hospitals and healthcare systems spend large sums on information technology without a clear return on investment. It appears to those providers that new and better information technology is just the right thing to do, without clearly identifying cost and quality benefits. It's now time for every information technology purchase to have a clear return on investment (ROI) analysis attached to it. If it doesn't provide a financial payback of less than so many years or achieve measurable quality improvement goals, then it should be questioned. Is that purchase adding true value for the patient? Would an uninsured patient be willing to pay for this new technology? Purchasing more and more computer technology requires hiring more highly paid technical workers to maintain it, which detracts from its cost benefit. Lean, value-added processes must come before adding more computer technology and automation. Still, if the new computer technology produces a truly desirable ROI and enables reaching quality goals, then it's desirable after internal processes have first been improved.

It's now nearly standard for a personal computer to be on every desk, just like a phone, and have a local area network connection, if not an Internet connection. There is enough computing power in each U.S. hospital to launch a Mars space mission and beyond! Each hospital now has a sophisticated Web site. Ask your information systems manager how many hits you receive per month on each part of your hospital's Web site. You may be surprised by the low utilization of parts of your Internet site that cost you dearly. Also, how fast and responsive is your Web site? Do users exit the Web site because it's just too slow? Would patients have willingly paid for its development? Is the Web site directly benefiting patients and employees, or could those expenditures have been more prudently deployed? Some Web contents, for example, job openings, are clearly value-added. Could your Web site be more spartan, providing just essential value-added information for patients and employees?

Speaking of Internet connections and e-mail, it is important that they be used appropriately for business purposes within an organization. Any company that thinks it's immune to internet abuse should take note of these survey statistics from the Spring 2003 *Technology Law Newsletter*[10]:

- 37 percent of employees said they surf the Web constantly at work.

- 8 percent of employees use workplace e-mail for personal use.

- 46 percent of online holiday shoppers make their purchases from work.

A recent audit of IRS employee usages of the Internet found that activities such as personal e-mail, online chats, shopping, and checking personal finances and stocks accounted for 51 percent of employees' time spent online! That's 51 percent of time people were supposed to have been doing value-added work! What percent of time do employees spend online at your organization doing non-value-added activities?

Software is commercially available that restricts personal Internet, chat, and e-mail usage.[11] Based on these statistics it would appear to be a good investment for any company, including hospitals and clinics. Internet and e-mail abuse is another example of significant waste in healthcare that is growing and that most providers aren't yet addressing.

Government relations

Some large hospitals/clinics have high-level government relations specialists on staff to study and help steer pending legislation. This is a type of overproduction. Again, it is not something most patients wish to pay for. What we need instead is a logical, national healthcare strategy and direction designed to increase quality and reduce cost.

24. Sequence work and standardize it

The father of lean production, Taiichi Ohno stated, "In the Toyota production system, sequencing of work and work standardization are done first. 'Efficient patient workflow' means that we provide defined value to the patient in each step of a process while the patient flows along. Moving the patient from place to place is in itself not continuous workflow but work forced to flow. Accomplishing as many steps as possible with minimal movement and transport between process steps is most efficient and constitutes 'continuous and efficient patient work flow.' In this way, most problem areas can be eliminated or improved."[12]

Once the work sequence has been improved and standardized, then additional improvements can follow by purchasing better equipment where justified. Purchasing new or better equipment is one way of improving work. "But, if equipment improvement comes first, work processes will never be improved," says Ohno. One will often find that even an old, well-maintained piece of equipment will deliver good service with a lean process that flows continuously. After sequencing and standardizing processes to achieve continuous flow, allow each department the opportunity to review the adequacy of their equipment and surrounding physical environment.

If it's clear that an improved instrument or piece of equipment or other physical change will significantly improve productivity, cost, or quality, then provide a method to accurately analyze, prioritize, and approve such purchases on an as needed or at least an annual basis. Do an ROI analysis on each request. Inadequate or faulty instruments, devices, and equipment, or other elements of the physical work environment can hamper other process improvement steps. Use the right tools and equipment and make them easily accessible. All too often, important instruments and equipment are not readily available or in proper working condition. Above all, however, sequence and standardize work to achieve lean production. Thirty years ago at the beginning of my career in healthcare, I believed that computers, automation, and new information systems were the ultimate solution for improving healthcare. Today I know that the *real* solution is to relentlessly pursue continuous process improvement. Computers and automation and other new purchases are secondary to first improving work processes.

In Appendix D, Jennifer Condel, Anatomic Pathology Team Leader at the University of Pittsburgh Medical Center Shadyside Hospital, and her colleagues present a wonderful case study of TPS in healthcare entitled "Error-Free Pathology: Applying Lean Production Methods to Anatomic Pathology." They show how the University of Pittsburgh Medical Center Shadyside Hospital uses Toyota continuous flow methods with the goal of reducing pathology process time from 48 hours to 24 hours (from obtaining the specimen to reporting the results). Credits are also due to Dr. Stephen S. Raab, MD, David T. Sharbaugh, and Karen Wolk Feinstein, PhD as detailed in Appendix D. A related article "Small Improvements Yield Big Results in Shadyside Pathology Lab" also appears in the August 2004 newsletter of the Pittsburgh Regional Healthcare Initiative (PRHI) Web site at http://prhi.org/newsletters.cfm. The online article was authored with the help of PRHI Communications Director Naida Grunden. The PRHI Web site at www.prhi.org contains numerous improvement examples that may be replicated by other healthcare providers.

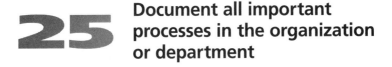

Document all important processes in the organization or department

It's important to document standardized processes to ensure continued conformance. It's not necessary to adopt rigorous ISO 9000–type process documentation, but at least document all major processes and all significant improvements using your organization's policy/ procedure format. Remember to include an up-to-date process flow-chart. Document in detail how a standardized process is supposed to be executed every time to achieve the desired level of cost and quality. Without this documentation, and a commitment to follow it consistently, the process will vary uncontrollably. Use the indicators on the scorecard discussed in step 2 to ensure that the new standard process is being effectively executed. In the next steps, we'll improve the standard process so that it functions with even higher quality and lower cost.

After making improvements to a process, update the policy/ procedure documentation. Use a scorecard to hold the gains and confirm you're doing so. Without a focused effort to hold the gains, a process will easily revert to prior variability, and hard-won improvements can be easily lost. Adopting ISO 9000 process documentation may be helpful in holding the gains, as there is a yearly audit to ensure that processes are being actually being performed according to the documented standards. Focus on standardizing process steps and maintaining those standards rather than reinventing the wheel each time to deal with situations. When staff change, ensure that the new staff are trained in and adopt the approved standards and documentation.

26 Implement and maintain continuous improvement

The Japanese word for continuous improvement is *kaizen*. This is what Toyota does every day to continuously improve cost and quality. These are small steps taken every day to improve quality and cost. Kaizen involves continuous process improvement, elimination of waste, inventory reduction through just-in-time kanban techniques, total productive maintenance of all instruments and equipment to minimize breakdowns, policy deployment so that all employees understand the basic strategic plan, an active employee suggestion system, and ongoing team activities to continuously improve both quality and cost.

Organizations should define the methods and tools to be used for improvement activities and include them in the quality and cost improvement manual and related training. Examples include:

- Identify each process owner. This is a simple but critical step that is often ignored. Identifying the process owner is the first step to improving the process since it immediately assigns responsibility and accountability for improvement.

- Educate the process owner about improvement methods.

- Define process boundaries.

- Establish functional and cross-functional improvement teams.

- Train the teams in improvement methods.

- Use tools such as diagrams, statistical techniques, and check sheets to improve.

- Map key processes using flowcharts.

- Measure the effectiveness and efficiency of the system and continually improve.

It may be necessary to reiterate several times between steps 25 and 26 to achieve a final standardized process. It may be necessary to first document a standardized process before being able to improve it using improvement techniques. After improvement, it will be necessary to redocument the newly improved standardized process. As continuous improvement occurs, these two steps of standardization and improvement may be repeated continuously until a desired standardized outcome is gradually achieved. Still, continuous improvement does not stop there. There is a relentless ongoing pursuit for perfection in the process.

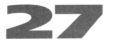 # Consider radical improvement where appropriate

As we've just learned, *kaizen* means continuous improvement. There is another Japanese word, *kaikaku,* which means radical improvement. Radical improvement may involve rearranging major processes in a single day with a doubling of productivity and a dramatic reduction in errors. This is similar to the concept of reengineering in the West. Often reengineering efforts stop at boundaries within the organization and consultants then collect their fees and leave. They fail to consider and improve the entire value stream for the patient or customer. They often treat employees as the enemy to be eliminated, which is contrary to our philosophy of respecting employees, helping develop them, and striving to retain them. Undertake reengineering efforts with great care and lots of open, honest communication. If good-performing staff are displaced, ensure that they have first preference for any open positions in the organization. Honor and respect their past contributions to the organization, and maintain a long-term view of their continuing future value to the organization.

28 Videotape each step of entire work process

Videotaping is best, but if it's not possible, at least still-photograph the steps from end to end to identify opportunities for improvement. An RIC then views the videotape repeatedly to identify alternatives for improvement and applies the organization's quality and cost improvement methods. This videotaping may reenergize the RIT or RICs if they are losing momentum.

Typically, expensive consultants are hired to observe departmental processes and suggest ways to improve their cost and quality. It is possible to train a subgroup of an RIC or a subgroup of the hospital's internal quality and cost improvement department to do process observations and videotaping, make recommendations to the department head, and report progress. It's a good idea to include the department head or supervisor and RIC members as ad hoc members of this team. This departmental observation team may observe non-value-added activities, waste in all its forms, excess inventory, idle equipment and facilities, and underutilized employees.

New approaches are needed to stop skyrocketing healthcare costs and to simultaneously improve quality. It is better to implement an observation team from within than to hire one-time consultants who will eventually leave. Doing even a major cost reduction/ quality improvement effort doesn't need to cost millions of dollars for consultants and be a one-time effort that will likely eventually evaporate. I am aware of several consultant-led quality and cost improvement engagements that did in fact cost several million dollars each and had transitory results. Improvement can and must be built into the organization. This can be done with a trained facilitator or two, one of whom may be the director of the existing internal quality and cost improvement department or a vice president, accompanied by the supporting structure described in Figure 3.1.

29 Use flowcharts to improve core processes

Core processes are the main customer value-added processes of the business. Flowchart these important processes. Flowcharting software such as Microsoft Visio may assist, but hand drawn flowcharts are adequate. A *core process* is defined as one of the primary processes the organization uses to achieve its mission or purpose. For example, the following are considered to be core processes for a hospital and need to be made as efficient as possible, as they represent the primary functions within the hospital. Each core process is labeled PVA if it is primarily patient value-added or BVA if it is primarily business value-added and not something a patient would normally choose to pay for.

- Admission (BVA)

- Emergency room treatment (PVA)

- All patient scheduling processes, for example, inpatient, outpatient (BVA)

- Outpatient treatment (PVA)

- Ancillary testing, for example, lab, x-ray (PVA)

- Surgical treatment (PVA)

- Medical treatment (PVA)

- Nursing care process (PVA)

- Therapy treatments (PVA)

- Medication process (PVA)

- Discharge (BVA)

- Billing and administration (BVA)

It is important to remove all non-valued-added steps and functions within these core processes as they represent waste. Ask yourself, "What would I, as a patient, be willing to pay for that step or activity or function?" Eliminate those steps or functions that do not provide direct value to the patient or the business. Some process steps or functions may not be value-added to the patient, but may be business value-added to the organization. They may be necessary for the organization to function appropriately. For example, the entire billing process and other administrative processes do not provide direct value to the patient, but are necessary for the organization to survive. Still, business value-added processes need to be minimized and probably also contain many non-value-added steps that can be eliminated. Patient value-added processes must be made more efficient or even possibly increased if the patient desires.

30 Use spaghetti diagrams to trace the path of a patient or product

A *spaghetti diagram* is a diagram of a department or facility that shows the actual path taken by a patient or product as it moves through a process. The spaghetti diagram will illustrate all the movement the patient or product makes within a process. All the starts, stops, and large distances traversed are sometimes very surprising.

Strive for a final spaghetti diagram that minimizes starts and stops, waits, and distances. It should show a continuous, direct, and efficient flow.

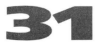 ## Measure process cycle times

In addition to making flowcharts and spaghetti diagrams of important processes, measure cycle times within processes. *Cycle time* may be defined as the total time it takes to complete a process step or a specific sequence of process steps. One can get a good sense of how well a process is working by just taking five to 10 cycle time measurements of each step in the process as well as for the entire process. This may not be statistically valid, but these observations will immediately give you a quick understanding of how well the process is working. If necessary, you can later do 30 to 100 cycle time measurements of each step to get more precise understanding. Often, the initial quick and dirty 5 to 10 measurements will point out obvious opportunities.

Implement quick changeovers within a process

A quick changeover allows a process to resume with little delay, maximizing available resources. Examples are operating room, emergency room, and cath lab room turnover times between cases; procedure room turnovers in other ancillary departments like x-ray, nuclear medicine, CT scan; lab draw cycle times between patients; and bed turnover time between patient departure and next patient arrival. Teach employees to distinguish between internal changeover times that create a pause in the process and external changeover times that can be done in parallel with the process without halting it. To achieve best success, employees should form a quick-changeover team led by an employee who has the best understanding of the changeover technology. They should set goals as a group to improve the changeover time by, for example, 50 percent.

Picture a pit crew in a NASCAR automobile race. It's amazing how fast they can now return a race car to the track. I'm sure it wasn't that way 50 years ago. Now, it may be a large crew where everyone knows their duties; it may use technology like quick-fill fuel cans/ systems, and lug wrenches that remove all the lug nuts from a wheel at the same time, and not just one such wrench but four working in parallel to change all four tires at once. Picture that type of pit crew commitment to turning over a cardiac surgery suite.

A goal-setting method that encourages efficient changeovers is to post a sign that lists the names of quick-changeover team members, the leader's name, and the time it last took to perform the changeover, as well as the target time. Hang the sign for all to see. When targets are achieved, the quick-changeover team performs demonstrations for other staff to see how it's done. Present an award or achievement certificate to the team that performs the demonstration.

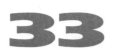

Challenge and work with your extended network of suppliers and partners

Help suppliers and partners improve. Treat them as an extension of your own business. Map the flow from suppliers and partners all the way through to patient discharge. Together, improve processes to achieve continuous flow between you and your partners. Set challenging targets. Create continuous flow of small lots (hours rather than days) of supplies and materials from vendors.

At a Toyota plant, there is less than an hour's worth of inventory next to each worker. This is made possible through the use of the continuous kanban supply system. Furthermore, suppliers deliver directly to the worker's station, sometimes hourly and certainly several times a day, with no inspection required. The inventory savings immediately fall to the bottom line. The lean assembler has no reserve stocks. A faulty shipment can be disastrous, but this almost never happens because the suppliers know what that can mean. And if a part is defective, the work team will immediately identify the cause to prevent a recurrence.

Toyota identifies a group of primary first-tier suppliers in which Toyota retains a minority financial interest. The first-tier suppliers use other second-tier suppliers that are completely independent. Certify suppliers based on defects per million, so that no inspection is required on receiving. If their defect rates are excessive, then transfer a portion of orders to other suppliers for a limited period of time until quality improves. Retain a cooperative relationship with all suppliers. Work with them as a team to continuously improve their processes and reduce their costs. Typically, Toyota uses a third to an eighth as many suppliers as traditional U.S. automakers. Toyota's technique of single sourcing supplies is not just a matter of simply selecting one supplier. It is rather the building of a long-term relationship based on a contract framework that encourages cooperation. Toyota works with the supplier to reduce the supply cost while maintaining the supplier's profit, or even allowing the supplier to receive an additional profit from a portion of any cost reduction achieved. The idea is for the lean assembler to work with the supplier so that they can become a lean supplier. This is a fundamental shift away from the power-based negotiating present in U.S. industries.

Some healthcare suppliers may be clinical partners that refer patients to you. Ensure that the referral process is simple, quick, seamless, and as smooth as possible. To the extent possible, transfer all demographic and insurance information and medical records from the partner so that you do not have to re-ask patient demographic and insurance questions. Expect that there will be no defects in the referral process and hold to this standard. Transfer information between information systems to help solve this problem or consider new technology such as smart ID cards that store patient information. Or, just ask the partner to provide a printout to the patient containing all current demographic and insurance information.

34 Automate processes to further improve quality and cost

Improve processes first. Simplify value-added steps, and eliminate all non-value-added steps. After processes have been manually improved and standardized, then it's time to automate. Remember, first simplify and eliminate, then automate. Do a careful cost–benefit analysis of any proposal for automation. Be sure you are improving quality and/or reducing costs. Otherwise question why you are automating. Don't automate just for the sake of automation.

First establish firm new goals for improved quality and cost. Beware of untested or "bleeding edge" technology that may cause extreme process disruptions. Use only reliable, time-tested technology. Be sure it is well-tested and verified before proceeding. Conduct thorough pilot tests under similar conditions. You may find that automation just isn't worth it when you consider the additional equipment cost and the ongoing cost of the labor and parts to maintain it. Adopt automation carefully in synch with your specific goals to improve processes, improve quality, and reduce cost. After thorough analysis, quickly implement well-tested technologies that will improve flow in your processes.

35 Learn from benchmark non-healthcare organizations

Emulate Toyota, Ritz Carlton Hotels, Wal-Mart, McDonalds, and Disney. Don't just watch what they do. Make a focused effort to do what they do and even improve upon that. Most of us are familiar with Wal-Mart. What can one learn from Wal-Mart? Some of the next points may not directly reduce cost, but do improve quality as perceived by the customer and do increase market share without the need for expensive marketing and advertising. K-Mart was near bankruptcy because of these customer-oriented practices Wal-Mart uses to increase quality and market share.

- Wal-Mart has a greeter who invariably says, "Welcome to Wal-Mart!" When did you last hear, "welcome" or when did you at least feel welcome as you entered a hospital?

- If you ask where something is located at Wal-Mart, an associate courteously takes you there without hesitation. Does that regularly happen in a hospital?

- Wal-Mart has a no-hassle price matching policy. If you can show any ad from a local store for the same item, it will match the price, no questions asked. Actually, Wal-Mart goes beyond simple price matching. It actually posts the ads from local competitors on a bulletin board near the main entrance. A customer need only look at all the local ads and then ask for a price match. Has any healthcare provider ever done price matching like that even though procedure costs vary greatly among providers? Have providers ever posted competitor's prices for easy comparison in a public area? I highly doubt it.

I once asked a healthcare provider to quote a price for a procedure, and after about 20 minutes I was given a handwritten scrap of paper with a wide range of costs written on it that I found difficult to understand. I wasn't impressed. I wouldn't have accepted that from an automobile body, brake, or muffler shop, but I was forced to accept it from the healthcare provider. As a customer, I did not feel I was well-served, and I would be delighted if in the future a health care provider were able to quickly provide accurate cost estimates for services.

- Wal-Mart has a no-hassle return policy if a customer is dissatisfied for any reason. I bought a jacket at Wal-Mart, and after a couple months the zipper stopped working. I brought it back and quickly and courteously received a new jacket, without any questions. Another time, I bought some cheese that was on sale at the Wal-Mart food store. When I got home, I noticed that it rang up on the register receipt at regular price. Since the store is only a couple blocks away from my home, I returned it later that afternoon. Wal-Mart didn't just refund the difference, but actually gave me the cheese for free as it was its own pricing error. If there was an error on a healthcare bill, would the provider just refund the difference, or something more than that, to compensate for the patient's trouble in calling attention to the error?

Also, if a healthcare procedure has some untoward outcome, like an infection, do healthcare providers promptly and courteously offer to refund the procedure cost or do follow-up procedures for free?

• I have been impressed by Wal-Mart's return policies, and lately I am wondering if its return policy ever disagrees with a customer's desires. I have begun to feel like testing the limits of its great customer service to see if it will disappoint rather than delight me as a customer. Most recently I bought a sealed package of six bars of hand soap, and found that I was allergic to it. Of course, I had to open and use a bar to find that out. I returned the unopened five bars with the broken cellophane packaging around them and explained that I was allergic to it. I explained that one bar was missing, since that was the one I used. Well, what do you think? Wal-Mart accepted the five returned bars and refunded me the full original price for the package of six. So I remain impressed with Wal-Mart's customer service policies to this day and must say I'm delighted.

• The outside signs at my local Wal-Mart say "Always low prices" above the discount store entrance. How many healthcare providers have a slogan like "Always low prices?" Many might say "Always rising prices at three to six times the rate of general inflation."

• Most Wal-Marts are open 24 hours a day and seven days a week. The sign above one entrance says "Always food center." That's called a "good access" strategy. The other local competing supermarket a few blocks away that closes at 10 PM had five cars in its parking lot at 9:30 PM while the Wal-Mart had about 50 cars in front of its food store and another 50 in front of the discount store. The competitor will be lucky to survive unless it quickly changes.

• Wal-Mart is clean and well-organized with pleasant music playing in the background. It has a large, well-lighted parking lot. It combines a discount store, food store, pharmacy, photo center, auto service center, gas station, and snack bar, along with several small boutique shops located at the main entrance. This is one-stop shopping. Customers can satisfy nearly all their shopping needs with one quick stop without undue waiting.

How often do patients have most of their needs filled with one stop? More commonly, a patient may not be able to see a particular physician for weeks and then may be referred to another physician who they must similarly wait for weeks to see, often at a different location. For example, patients in Boston wait, on average, more than a month to see medical specialists, the longest wait in a survey of 15 major cities. The shortest wait of eight to 15 days was in Washington, DC.[13] How many physicians and hospitals have open access appointment systems that can give a patient an appointment on the very day they call? How often do you hear or read about emergency rooms packed with patients waiting hours to be seen? In April 2002, the Associated Press reported that one in three hospitals is diverting ambulances due to overcrowding in their emergency rooms. This is an example of "poor access" strategies for healthcare services.

• If you get your car's oil changed at Wal-Mart, workers will also vacuum the interior and wash the windshield. This is an example of giving a customer more than they expect. This strategy will often delight a customer and encourage their return. How often do patients receive services that delight them and encourage them to return?

• As I finish the checkout at Wal-Mart, the cashier may say, "Thank you, Robert" after observing my name on my credit or debit card. How often do hospital employees call patients by their names, or do they more often treat patients as numbers? Customer service training should be required for all new healthcare employees and periodically refreshed for existing employees. Ritz Carlton hotels, for example, train every new employee for days to become ladies and gentlemen before they even begin their job.

And, what can hospitals learn from McDonald's? McDonald's has become an icon of American culture, almost like Coca-Cola. How did they become so successful? It all started over 50 years ago when Ray Kroc traveled to San Bernardino, California, to learn why a small hamburger stand had just ordered 10 of the milk shake mixing machines that he was selling. They must have been doing something special to need this big order.

• What Ray Kroc saw in San Bernardino in 1955 was Richard and Maurice McDonald making hamburgers more efficiently than anyone else using their new "Speedee Service System." Ray believed he could replicate this best practice in his home state of Illinois and other parts of the U.S., and McDonald's was born. Retired coaches can remember taking a busload of basketball players to McDonald's in the 1960s and ordering 100 hamburgers and 50 or 60 orders of fries, and amazingly getting their order in about 10 minutes. And, the kids liked it.

• Ray Kroc insisted his McDonald's restaurants look the same, and that all staff follow the same procedures across the country to produce the same high-quality product at an affordable price. Now people go to McDonald's from Boston to Beijing because they know what they are going to get. They simply want reliable, predictable, high-quality, and reasonably priced products and services—the same thing that hospital patients want.

• Early on, McDonald's listened to their customers. In the 1950s and 1960s, automobile ownership was rising fast and more mothers were working. McDonald's filled these customers' needs for easy access and speedy service and at the same time catered to the tastes of America. Is healthcare adequately responding today to its customer needs?

• What have been the results of standardization, speed, reasonable cost, and meeting customer's needs with predictable service quality at McDonald's? The small chain that started in the 1950s now boasts over 30,000 restaurants serving 50 million people a day. McDonald's is still a high-performing business example today, with a 55 percent jump in profits in 2004 to $2.3 billion. They have adjusted to the times with healthier salad options and have launched a campaign to teach children about the benefits of healthy eating and exercise. Hospitals and other healthcare providers can similarly become successful by standardizing their business practices, streamlining their operations, and simply listening to the needs of their customers.

36 Learn from other benchmark healthcare organizations

Learn from Baldrige Award finalists and winners. What is the Malcolm Baldrige National Quality Award? The Baldrige Award is annually given by the president of the United States to businesses— manufacturing and service, small and large—and to education and healthcare organizations that apply and are judged to be outstanding in seven areas: leadership, strategic planning, customer and market focus, information and analysis, human resource focus, process management, and business results.

From 1987 to 2002 there have been 51 Baldrige Award recipients. The Baldrige Award for Healthcare was established in 1999. Forty-two Baldrige Healthcare applications have been submitted since its inception. In 2002, the Franciscan Sisters of Mary Health Care (SSMHC) based in St. Louis, Missouri, received the first Baldrige Award for Healthcare. SSMHC is composed of 21 hospitals and three nursing homes located throughout the Midwest. Any healthcare organization can learn from SSMHC and use the same Baldrige criteria and application to improve, even if it's not submitted.[14]

In a recent press release, SSMHC stated, "Since 1999, SSMHC has exceeded its charity care goal of contributing a minimum of 25 percent of its operating margin (before deductions) from the prior year. Currently, in excess of 33 percent of SSMHC's previous year's operating margin (before deductions) is used to provide care to people who cannot pay." This is an example for every hospital in America to emulate. Possibly Congress should consider a law that would require each hospital to similarly contribute a certain percentage of it's operating margin (profit) or cash reserves to charity care in order to maintain its not-for-profit corporate status. This would help provide some relief to the growing numbers of uninsured.

Similarly, Baptist Health Care (BHC) of Pensacola, Florida, is nationally recognized as one of the nation's truly outstanding healthcare organizations for both staff and patients. BHC is ranked among the fifteen best companies to work for in the United States, according to *Fortune* magazine's annual "100 Best Companies to Work for in America" list. The companies on this list are selected from a large national pool of candidate organizations and ranked based principally on how a random selection of employees responded to a survey that measures the quality of their workplace culture. Completing the patient–employee connection, BHC has been in the top one percent in perceived patient satisfaction, from research conducted among hospitals nationwide, for the past five years. Today, BHC has one of the lowest annual hospital staff turnover rates in the nation (just over 14 percent) and one of the highest levels of employee morale for any company in any industry.[15]

Notice, however, that even this achievement of 14 percent annual staff turnover still means that about one in seven employees is leaving

BHC annually. That still implies large rehiring costs, which aren't patient value-added. More improvement is needed. Imagine what levels of turnover other less successful hospitals are experiencing.

How does the Baldrige Award differ from ISO 9000?

The purpose, content, and focus of the Baldrige Award and ISO 9000 are very different. The Baldrige Award was created by Congress in 1987 to enhance U.S. competitiveness. The award program promotes quality awareness, recognizes quality achievements of U.S. organizations, and provides a vehicle for sharing successful strategies. The Baldrige Award criteria focus on results and continuous improvement. They provide a framework for designing, implementing, and assessing a process for managing all business operations.

ISO 9000 is a series of three international standards, first published in 1987 by the International Organization for Standardization (ISO), Geneva, Switzerland and updated and revised periodically. Companies can use the standards to help determine what is needed to maintain an efficient quality conformance system. For example, the standards describe the need for an effective quality system, for ensuring that measuring and testing equipment is calibrated regularly, and for maintaining an adequate record-keeping system. ISO 9000 certification determines whether a company complies with its own quality system.

Overall, ISO 9000 registration covers less than 10 percent of the Baldrige Award criteria, since it provides little encouragement for continuous improvement. Organizations with advanced quality systems can still consider it, especially for its yearly audit of standardized processes. Table 3.2 further compares Baldrige and ISO 9000 approaches.

37 ## Learn from the Institute for Healthcare Improvement

In addition to the preceding two steps, refer to the Institute for Healthcare Improvement (IHI) as a valuable source for cost reduction and quality improvement ideas (www.ihi.org). IHI hosts free

Internet e-mail groups on topics such as "Idealized Design of Clinical Office Practices" that can be invaluable in helping improve healthcare quality and cost. IHI's publications and collaboratives also tackle many of the current problems within healthcare. IHI sponsors several initiatives that focus on specific core problems. Some of these IHI initiatives may be independently pursued. However, pursuing IHI's individual initiatives does not take the place of building a permanent internal structure for continuous quality improvement and cost reduction as described in this book.

38 Hold onto the gains you've achieved!

All too often, consultants or improvement projects start, become successful, and, after a couple years, the gains evaporate. Consultants leave and gains slowly disappear. More than once, I have observed the gains from multimillion dollar engagements dissipate within a few years. Or, improvement teams work hard to achieve meaningful gains, and then when they disband or change their focus, their gains slowly disappear. So a critical and often overlooked step is to put measures in place to hold your gains permanently.

This may mean continuing to monitor the improvement via your finance or quality and cost improvement department, or via a periodic scorecard that includes monitoring measures. Better yet, permanently build your improvements into the new process. It may mean documenting a new standard procedure and posting it at the job station. It may mean training each new employee in that standard procedure as they start the job. It may mean a periodic review, audit, or training update to ensure that the standard procedure is being followed. Good documentation of newly improved methods and procedures using the organizations policy and procedure format is important to maintain any improvement. It is a good idea for employees to review process documentation at least annually and to discuss any deviations with their team leader (supervisor). The last thing you want is for gains to slowly evaporate or for a new team to come along a couple years later, misunderstand the situation, and change the procedure back to a less effective one.

4

A Capsule Summary of a Lean Toyota-Like Production System for Healthcare

What follows is a capsule summary of the characteristics of a lean Toyota-like production system that we are trying to implement in healthcare. At the core of a lean TPS is respect for the employee. It is the core value around which lean TPS is built. It means encouraging employees to make improvements to their jobs and the organization, and respecting everyone's opinions. It means taking a long-term view of their employment and doing everything in your power to retain good-performing employees and, if necessary, deploy them elsewhere in the organization where they can continue to provide good value.

Beyond the core of respect for employees are the following key activities within lean TPS:

1. Embed a permanent structure for cost and quality improvement in the organization. This is a most important and critical action. This structure will automatically and relentlessly function every day to continuously improve healthcare quality and cost. It begins with a constant, clear, and visible commitment from every member of the organization's leadership, starting with the CEO, to continually improve quality and reduce costs. It utilizes small Toyota-style work teams of three to eight cross-trained employees with a team leader who facilitates and

shares in their tasks. It uses a group leader (that is, manager or supervisor) over multiple teams, all totaling up to approximately 60 employees. It includes board-sponsored strategic goals and teams to achieve those strategic cost and quality goals in a timely manner. It includes an RIT of all managers and supervisors to jump-start the lean TPS. Then RICs of volunteer employees meet periodically on company time to continually improve quality and cost. Ask each employee in an RIC quality circle to submit two suggestions for cost and quality improvement per month, and reward them appropriately. Later, ask every employee in the organization to submit two suggestions per month. RICs evaluate the suggestions related to their areas.

2. Establish an improvement plan with goals accomplished by specific people and completion dates. Include in that plan the benchmark targets that you are going to achieve.

3. Establish an award/recognition/reward/gain-sharing program to encourage all to participate in cost and quality improvement. The hospital board approves this program to support its strategic objectives. Thank people publicly and repeatedly for their good contributions. Express sincere appreciation.

4. Create a simple, easy-to-understand quality and cost improvement manual to educate every employee.

5. Educate every employee about the organization's strategic plan, and be sure they document their own personal goals and understand how they contribute to the strategic plan.

6. Create continuous flow. This means that the patient will easily move through the system with no waits and delays. The patient will immediately pull needed value-added activities to themselves as they move through the system of care and treatment. Use tools like direct observation teams, videotaping, flowcharts, value stream maps, spaghetti diagrams, and so on, to achieve continuous flow. Measure and continuously improve cycle times of process steps.

7. Sequence work and standardize it. This means having a standard best-practice way of doing each process step, clearly documenting it, and preferably having that documentation clearly visible at the location where the process step is performed. Train each employee to perform the process steps in the standardized fashion.

8. Implement quick changeovers of rooms, staff, and equipment within process steps to minimize downtime.

9. Create quality in station. This means that each worker at a process step creates no errors or defects, and the same worker who is performing a process step also does inspections to ensure quality. Very little or, preferably, no follow-up inspection is needed, and no defects are passed to the next step.

10. Create a system for any employee to immediately stop/fix a defective process by immediately informing the team leader (supervisor) and/or group leader (manager) by personal contact, phone, page, or other immediate signal. Correct the process immediately so that the defect will not occur again.

11. Constantly eliminate waste in all its forms. This means eliminating all non-value-added steps that an uninsured patient would not choose to pay for. Define true value from the point of view of the patient (customer).

12. Reduce inventory and supplies to minimum levels that are still safe. This means providing inventory and supplies in small quantities when and where they are needed. Recall that two hours of inventory is typical in TPS. Certainly organizations should avoid having weeks of inventory. Kanban signals provide inventory and supplies to processes at the rate that those processes use them up.

13. Create a visual workplace. This means that a casual observer can see all the work being done. This entails a reduction in private office space so the value-added activities of each employee are visible. It also means having needed equipment, instruments, inventory, and supplies well-organized, visible, and easily accessible to employees.

14. Challenge and work with your extended network of suppliers and partners. Help them improve with you.

15. Hold your gains. Build your improvements into a well-documented standard process. Use a simple periodic scorecard to ensure that your hard-earned improvements do not evaporate. Enlist your finance department and your cost and quality improvement department to sustain your improvements and ensure that they are built to last.

16. After focusing first on internal process improvements and achieving them, then consider additional automation to further improve quality and cost. First simplify, then improve processes, and afterward automate. Be sure to do a cost–benefit analysis on every new capital purchase.

5

A Short To-Do List to Nationally Improve U.S. Healthcare Cost and Quality

1. Begin now to implement the 38 steps to improve healthcare quality and cost as presented in this book. Permanently build the structure for cost and quality improvement into your organization, as shown in Figure 3.1 on page 39, and maintain it. Eliminate all forms of waste and non-value-added activities. Focus on doing only value-added steps that an uninsured patient would actually choose to pay for. Continuously and relentlessly pursue quality and cost improvement. Certain hospitals in the United States are much more efficient than others. Copy other known best practices within the United States and worldwide (for example, Baldrige winners and other healthcare and non-healthcare benchmark performers).

2. Write your senators and representative and lobby for national, ideally designed hospitals and clinic demonstration sites. Our government should support even just one U.S. hospital system and clinic becoming a demonstration site of what can be achieved in highest quality and lowest cost. This demonstration project might be sponsored by IHI and supported by other quality and lean production experts. Encourage the use of industrial engineers and process improvement engineers to help improve healthcare just as they have helped Toyota and other companies improve. Many like myself would welcome the opportunity to participate. Create clear incentives to reduce cost and improve quality. Our government could then

form a national team to replicate the results of the demonstration site to other interested healthcare providers throughout the United States.

Alternatively, the American Hospital Association (AHA) or the Voluntary Hospital Association (VHA) could help sponsor or replicate demonstration sites. If a demonstration site is not likely to be sponsored at a national level, then lobby for your state government or state hospital association to sponsor or promote it. If that's unlikely, then strive for your own healthcare system to achieve demonstration site status so that others may see and emulate what you and your team have achieved. Then all other healthcare providers would be able to achieve similar world-class levels of quality and low cost. If voluntary improvement is not forthcoming, then state or national legislation to improve cost and quality will be necessary. Then there will be hope for the United States to achieve better than its current World Health rank of 37th in health system performance, without spending almost twice as much per capita on healthcare as any other nation in the world.

3. Stay tuned to changes and direction of national healthcare policy. Support new initiatives to reduce the 45 million uninsured in the United States and clamor for reduced healthcare costs. Lobby to reduce non-value-added activities, administrative costs, defects, medical errors, and waste. Support a system that improves access to the underserved. Support the importation of cheaper pharmaceutical drugs. As we are the only developed country in the world without national health insurance, carefully evaluate and consider that option, or at least consider a single-payer system like Maine.

4. Write your senators and representatives and lobby for completion of a certificate of need (CON) prior to any major new healthcare capital expenditure. This will help reduce growing duplication of equipment, services, and construction. If a national CON process is not likely, then at least lobby to implement a CON process within your state. Too often local city or county officials face decisions about choosing construction projects between volatile health care competitors, which is a competitive decision they should not have to face.

5. Ask for a healthcare scorecard for your community. The United Way organization appears to be supporting and making these cards available online.[1] Work with United Way and similar organizations to use and expand these scorecards to improve the status of healthcare in your community and region. Ask the board members of your local healthcare providers what they are doing by when to improve community health status indicators.

6. It's time for all U.S. healthcare providers to rapidly reduce cost and improve quality by implementing the lean production steps described in this book. Implementing lean production is an effective strategy to achieve value and quality in healthcare. Quality healthcare may then be more affordable for all.

Appendix A
Automaker Benchmarks

Comparing the best

Key productivity and other operating measures for leading assembly plants run by major automakers in the United States:

Automaker	Toyota	Honda	Nissan	GM	Ford	Chrysler
Plant location	Georgetown, Ky.	East Liberty, Ohio	Smyrna, Tenn.	Lansing Grand River, Mich.	Kansas City, Ka.	Toledo, Ohio
Products	Toyota Camry, Avalon, Sienna, Camry Solara convertible	Honda Civic, Element	Nissan Altima, Frontier, Xterra	Cadillac CTS sedan	Ford Escape, Mazda Tribute, Ford F-150 pickup	Jeep Liberty
2002 assembly employment	4,849	2,327	3,632	749	5,563	2,307
2002 output (in units)	490,618	222,742	409,806	47,072	518,137	225,703
Labor hours per vehicle	22.81 ('01) 20.85 ('02)	19.20 ('01) 21.43 ('02)	17.92 ('01) 16.83 ('02)	32.35 ('02) Plant not in operation ('01)	Escape, Tribute line: 22.54 ('01) 22.1 ('02); F-150, Blackwood line: 24.88 ('01) 24 ('02)	26.11 ('01) 24.02 ('02)
Capacity utilization rate* *Rate over 100 percent indicates plant ran on overtime*	94% ('01) 104% ('02)	97% ('01) 91% ('02)	85% ('01) 94% ('02)	Plant not in operation ('01) 57% ('02)	Escape, Tribute line: 125% ('01) 124% ('02); F-150, Blackwood line: 112% ('01) 123% ('02)	102% ('01) 122% ('02)
Initial quality *Problems per 100 cars in first 90 days of ownership*	Camry/Solara 110; Avalon 145; Sienna 123	Civic 121; Element 134	Altima 130; Frontier 151; Xterra 174	CTS 88	Escape 141; Tribute 151; F-150 117	Jeep Liberty 145

Intangibles

Toyota	Honda	Nissan	GM	Ford	Chrysler
• Has consistently built the popular Toyota Camry, among the most profitable, high-quality vehicles in Toyota lineup. • Has low absenteeism. • Has managed to overcome loss of key managers to rivals in recent years. • First Toyota plant in North America equipped with new welding system, the Global Body Line. • Consistently among most-utilized plants in U.S.	• Relied on overtime to prepare for Element launch, cope with West Coast strike by dock workers, which caused two down days. • Still consistently among most-utilized plants in U.S. • Has low absenteeism.	• Relies on high degree of automation in body shop, where steel skeleton is welded and assembled. • Also relies heavily on delivery of parts in sequence as needed, which eliminates excessive stockpiles. • Low absenteeism.	• Latest model of GM's manufacturing blueprint. • New plant and all-new product in 2002. • Very successful launch, met launch and quality targets. • One-shift operation. • Now builds Cadillac SRX SUV and preparing to build next generation STS sedan. • Cooperative, dedicated work force and labor union.	• Lincoln Blackwood output shelved in August 2002. • Ford's most productive pickup truck plant, despite higher, more complicated mix of content featured on trucks assembled in Kansas City. • One of Ford's most-utilized factories. Loyal, dedicated, focused, and cooperative workforce and labor union.	• Newest Chrysler plant and already among automaker's most-flexible plants, with ability to build diesel and right-hand drive versions of Liberty. • Slated for new expansion that will provide flexibility to build additional light truck products for Jeep.

*Rate over 100 percent indicates plant ran on overtime. Note: Mercedes-Benz and BMW do not participate in Harbour and Associates study; Civic and Camry quality scores include models assembled at other plants; plants selected through a variety of expert sources, automakers. Toyota's Georgetown plan stopped building the Sienna minivan in December 2002. *Sources:* Harbour and Associates, J.D. Power and Associates. *Source:* Reproduced with permission of *The Detroit News.*

Appendix B

Children's Hospital and Regional Medical Center Emergency Department Patient Flow—Rapid Process Improvement (RPI)

Application of Toyota Production System Principles of Continuous Flow and Pull

Credits to: George A. Woodward, MD, MBA, Larry Godt, Michele Girard, Kelly Fisher, Shaughna Feeley, Margaret Dunphy, Barb Bouché

PROBLEM STATEMENT

In early 2004, the Emergency Department (ED) at Children's Hospital and Regional Medical Center in Seattle, Washington, began a continuous performance improvement process in order to address the following issues:

- An inefficient and noncentralized model of care

- An increase in the ED overall patient Length of Stay (see Figure B.1)

- An increase in problem scores from the Family Experience Survey

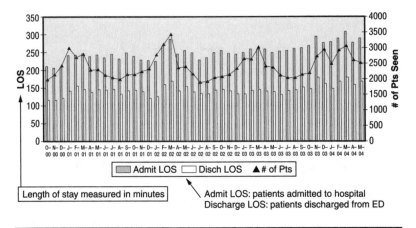

Figure B.1 Length of stay.

- Communication issues with the Referring Provider community

- Issues with continuum of care between community providers and hospital managment

Specifically, the ED wanted to:

- Improve the quality of care for patients based on data from the Family Experience Survey

- Improve efficiency of care, while decreasing waste in the system

- Improve communications with our Referring Community Physicians

- Ensure medical information capture between community, ED, and hospital providers

- Decrease ED patient length of stay

In addition, the ED would be moving into a new facility in 2007, and there was a desire to make corresponding improvements for the new facility.

INTERVENTION

A four-day RPI workshop was held in July 2004 in which the ED designed a new model of care. The ED implemented the work cell model in early December 2004 to provide more focused care, including the following elements:

1. Work cells called "pods (or zones)" were created. See Figure B.2.

   • Complex, Medium, and Fast pods/zones were created, based on historical and anticipated patient complexity and available supervision qualifications. Each pod/zone was staffed with an appropriate ratio of nurses, MDs, and Care Coordinators to treat the measured (and projected) volume of patients and required interventions in these pods. Staff such as Social Workers and Child Life Specialists were appropriately scheduled and located so as to provide a shared resource to all "pods."

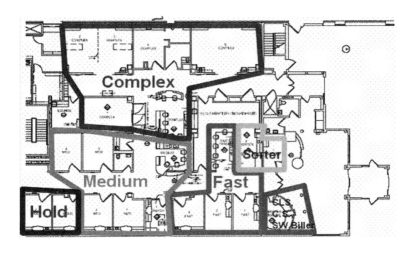

Figure B.2 New emergency department "pod design."

- A "pull" system was implemented that allowed for a better balance of patient demand to resource capability. As patients arrive in the ED, a provider completes a minimal intake to sort the patients based on acuity and assign them to a pod. ED related services and supplies are rapidly pulled to the ED patient based on their healthcare needs and associated orders.

- The design and location of the Fast, Medium, and Complex pods enable improved flow through the ED for patients and families. Teams of providers comprising the appropriate mix of disciplines work in assigned pods to facilitate the needed care for patients assigned to the pods.

2. Communications changes.

- A communication center was constructed and a Communication Specialist role was established to coordinate all incoming referrals, ED Team and in-hospital medical communications regarding expected or current patients, communication with and to Primary Care Providers (PCPs) regarding patient disposition and follow-up, as well as a notification system for when patients do not arrive as expected. This position is staffed 24/7 by an RN with additional communications training.

- An automated phone system was created to allow callers to choose the option that best fits their needs, including an option for the new communication center that coordinates all incoming communications from PCPs and medical transport teams en route to the ED.

3. Created a new patient chart for the ED. This "Uni-Form" combines both nurse and physician charting areas and replaces the multiple charting forms for patients.

During the first three months of implementation, the ED collected data to measure improvement in several key areas. This included measuring patient and staff satisfaction as well as ED length of stay. See Figures B.3 and B.4.

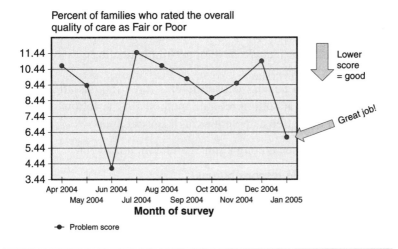

Figure B.3 Percent of families who rated the overall quality of care as fair or poor.

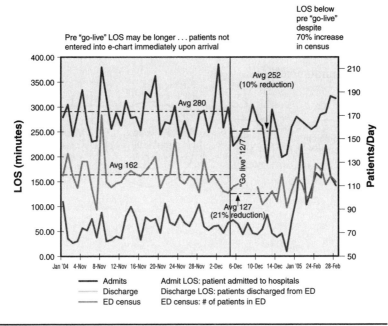

Figure B.4 Reduction in ED length of stay.

FOLLOW-UP ACTIONS

Upcoming actions include developing/implementing reliable methods as described below.

The ED team began Focused Events three months after implementation aimed at setting reliable methods in the following areas, which were identified as potential high-impact areas:

- Work balance among clinical and nonclinical staff

- Nursing role responsibilities

- Tasks assigned to Intake and Triage RNs

- Paperwork flow

- Lobby management

- Environmental Services support

- 5S projects

- Internal ED admission process

- Weekly Audits

- Communications

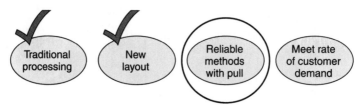

Appendix C

5S Catches on at the VA Pittsburgh Health System

(Sort, Set in order, Shine, Standardize, Sustain)

Credits to: VA Pittsburgh Healthcare System
Ellesha McCray, RN, Team Leader
Michael Moreland, CEO
Naida Grunden, Communications Director
Pittsburgh Regional Healthcare Initiative

Every business would like to improve productivity, reduce defects, meet deadlines, and provide everyone with a safer place to work. Yet in a complex hospital, making these kinds of major improvements might seem next to impossible.

At the 4 West Learning Unit at the VA Pittsburgh Healthcare System, staff discovered a relatively simple, rapid, low-cost, low-tech way of making these improvements. It's called 5S.

A LITTLE HISTORY

Before World War II, many American businesses had codified the idea that a clean workplace is a productive workplace. In America, by and large the idea remained in manuals, without being translated to the workplace. As Americans helped the Japanese reconstruct their industries after the war, they brought their ideas, and found the Japanese to be ready students. Before long, the Western idea of the orderly and productive workplace became tied to the Eastern idea of deep respect for the worker's well-being and morale. Out of this blend of philosophies came a technique for creating the orderly workplace, a technique directed not by a distant manager, but by the esteemed worker.

WHAT ARE THE FIVE S's?

The name, "5S," refers to a sequence of steps that translate approximately as follows:

Sort. Remove all items from the workplace that are not needed for current operations. A crowded workplace is hard to work in and costly to maintain.

Set in order. Arrange needed items so that they are easy to use. Label them so that they're easy to find, clean, and put away. This degree of order improves communication and reduces the frustration of wasted time and motion.

Shine. Clean the floors, walls, and equipment. When things are kept in top condition, when someone needs to use something, it is always ready. In a hospital environment, cleanliness is extremely important to staff member and patient alike.

Standardize. By integrating the first three steps into everyday work, "backsliding" is eliminated.

Sustain. If the rewards for keeping order outweigh the rewards for going back to the old way of doing things, people will make orderliness a habit.

PRACTICING 5S AT THE VA

About a year ago, the workers on 4 West, the inpatient surgical unit, took a long look at their equipment storage room. It looked like a typical storage room in any American hospital—a mix of often- and seldom-used equipment, stored in no particular order. It took time to find equipment, and it was difficult to walk around in the room. Items relying on recharged batteries were not always plugged in.

It wasn't clear where or in what condition things were supposed to be stored.

Following a deliberate process over a few weeks, staff members on 4 West were able to reduce the inventory in the room, while still maintaining access to what they needed when they needed it. About $20,000 worth of seldom used equipment was freed up for use in other areas of the hospital.

Signs clearly denote where each piece of equipment is to be stored, how it is to be cleaned, whether it is to be plugged in, and so on. The visual cues leave no doubt about the expectations.

Since the 5S, the room and equipment have been maintained in sparkling clean condition with little problem. Since cleaning is built into the work itself, backsliding is minimal.

So well has the equipment storage room worked that staffers on other units are now learning 5S. In short order, units on the fifth and sixth floors are organizing their storage rooms according to the principles.

"It's not just a matter of cleaning out your closet," says Peter Perreiah, PRHI's team leader at the VA. "It's about honoring the worker with a clean, safe environment, and honoring patients with equipment that's always clean and ready."

5S CATCHES ON

When she saw the equipment storage room on 4 West, Shedale Pinnix-Tindall, Nurse Manager on 6 West, thought it could work in her unit as well. Nobody asked her to do it. But she and Marianne Allen, 6 West Charge Nurse, asked for help and soon got started.

"Who could be against this? Having the storage areas orderly like this really saves time and frustration. It's better for patients," says Shedale, "and it's not hard to keep it this way."

Says Environmental Aide, John R. Finkley, "Since we did the 5S on 4 West, we can get what we need easily and quickly for every patient. There's no guessing. You just open the door and go right to the item. I find that I spend less time cleaning that room, so there's more time to clean every piece of equipment thoroughly. It's all part of the routine now."

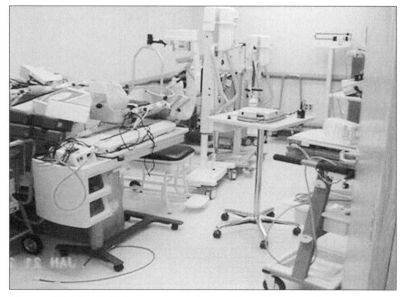

Figure C.1 Typical storage room in any American hospital.

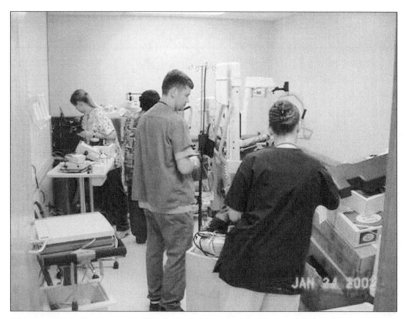

Figure C.2 Crew at VA Pittsburgh Health System amid the 5S process.

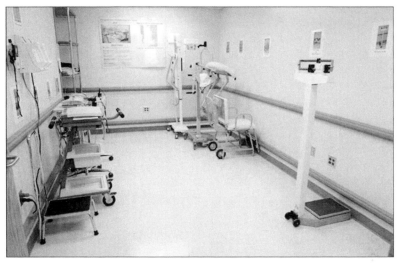

Figure C.3 Completed project. Wall posters visually delineate what goes where, how to clean and store.

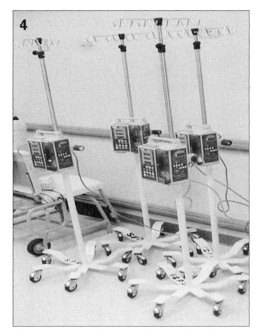

Figure C.4 Adequate electrical outlets mean equipment is always charged.

Appendix D

Error-Free Pathology: Applying Lean Production Methods to Anatomic Pathology

Jennifer L. Condel, BS, SCT(ASCP)MT,[a,*] David T. Sharbaugh, CPA,[b] Stephen S. Raab, MD[a]

[a]Department of Pathology, University of Pittsburgh Medical Center, Shadyside Hospital, Cancer Pavilion, 3rd Floor, 5150 Centre Avenue, Pittsburgh, PA 15232, USA
[b]University of Pittsburgh Medical Center, Presbyterian Shadyside Hospital, 5230 Centre Avenue, Pittsburgh, PA 15232, USA

By definition, "lean" refers to thin or sparse. In business, this word may have a negative connotation. The idea of "trimming the fat" or streamlining usually evokes the elimination of jobs. Employees therefore do not favor such techniques. At Toyota Motor Company, however, employees embrace "lean" as a work philosophy. This work ethic has developed through trial and error and evolved into the successful business practice known as the Toyota Production System (TPS). Lean methods, which include Six Sigma, strive to eliminate waste from a system. How this aim is accomplished varies among different methods, but one of the ultimate goals is a system that generates zero defects or errors.

This work was supported by the Jewish Healthcare Foundation, the Agency for Healthcare Research and Quality, and the University of Pittsburgh School of Medicine.

* Corresponding author.
E-mail address: condeljl@upmc.edu (J. L. Condel).

doi:10.1016/j.cll.2004.07.001 labmed.theclinics.com

Is error-free pathology possible? The authors think it is. If we do not challenge the current system and strive toward zero errors by experimentation, how will we know what is possible? This article is intended to share the authors' experiences in applying a lean production method to their anatomic pathology department, not only to reduce pathology errors to zero but to change a "blame culture" to one in which frontline staff members become effective problem solvers and the source of system improvements.

THE EVOLUTION OF LEAN

The phenomenon of lean business practice has drawn considerable attention over the last decade as a result of changing economics and customer demand. These same issues were the roots of the development of lean production after World War II, when Henry Ford's revolutionary manufacturing process of automobile mass production was practiced. The evolution of "lean" thinking may be traced through several generations of the Toyoda family. "They were innovators, they were pragmatic idealists, they learned by doing, and they always believed in the mission of contributing to society. They were relentless in achieving their goals . . . and they were leaders who led by example."[1]

An early example of lean thinking in the Toyoda family can be seen in the late 1800s, in the case of a carpenter and inventor named Sakichi Toyoda who designed wooden looms for weaving. Because the original design was labor-intensive, he strove to improve the looms for the women who used them. By 1926, Sakichi Toyoda had started the Toyoda Automatic Loom Works and successfully automated the loom using a steam engine. He is also credited with designing a mechanism by which the loom would automatically stop if a thread broke, thereby highlighting a problem. This practice of building quality into work, referred to as jidoka, enabled workers to perform value-added work and saved them from wasting time by watching machines work. From the root of this invention, jidoka became one of the two pillars of the lean production system known as TPS.[1]

In the early 1900s, an American named Henry Ford who was also interested in eliminating non-valued-added work created the cost-efficient process known as mass production for one style of automobile, the Model T. By incorporating people, materials, and machines in a continuous workflow design, Ford created cost-efficiency through simplicity: he synchronized the repetitive nature of tasks at each workstation, where only the materials needed were consumed.[2]

The Toyoda family advanced into the automotive industry when Sakichi Toyoda challenged his son Kiichiro to build an automobile business. Kiichiro Toyoda, a mechanical engineer, eventually built the Toyota Automotive Company and developed the idea of a "just-in-time" approach to work. This second pillar of TPS actually arose from Kiichiro Toyoda's trip to the United States, where he studied Ford's River Rouge automobile plant in Michigan and observed the replenishment system practiced in American supermarkets. The kanban replenishment system used in TPS is modeled after this process of "replacing products on the shelves just in time as the customers purchased them."[1] Kiichiro Toyoda's success was overshadowed after World War II; in 1948, he was faced with trying to prevent the company from going into bankruptcy as a result of overwhelming inflation. Toyoda's philosophy was not to fire employees under these circumstances. But his cost-cutting measures were inadequate, and he resigned as president, taking full responsibility for what he believed was his failure. Amazingly, other employees followed his lead and left voluntarily for the betterment of the company.

Kiichiro Toyoda continued to support the automobile industry by giving his cousin Eiji Toyoda, also a mechanical engineer, the task of establishing a "car hotel" (large parking garage) for a research laboratory. Toyota and other firms owned the "car hotel" for the purpose of supporting the small group of individuals who could still afford cars.[1] Eiji Toyoda researched the needs and supplies of the Toyota plant and ultimately became the president and chairman of Toyota.

MANUFACTURING COMPANY

Returning from a visit to Ford's Michigan plant in 1950, Eiji Toyoda gave Taiichi Ohno, a plant manager at that time, the task of "catching up with Ford's productivity."[1] Taiichi Ohno, Eiji Toyoda, and his managers spent 12 weeks studying the American plants. They observed what they believed were many system flaws and sources of waste, including disorganization and overhead as a result of excess inventory and large equipment needs. Taiichi Ohno was, however, impressed with Henry Ford's design of a continuous workflow assembly line that incorporated work standardization processes. Toyota's resources, unlike Ford's, were limited, and Taiichi Ohno knew Toyota needed to be able to produce small quantities of a variety of quality cars at the lowest cost in the shortest amount of time.

After World War II, customer demands changed and focused on variety. The American Big Three (Chrysler, General Motors, and Ford) responded to this change in demand by dismantling their original continuous flow design and switching to a process in which each portion of the assembly line functioned as an independent continuous flow entity. Taiichi Ohno viewed this form of mass production as introducing waste into the system. The process became more complex, requiring additional resources, and therefore was not an efficient way to meet the varied customer demands and maintain low production costs. Adopting Henry Ford's original workflow design, "a design that promoted efficiency by allowing work to flow continuously from beginning to end and by having it consume at every point only the resources needed to advance one unit of output one step further toward completion,"[3] Taiichi Ohno began to apply his learning to the shop floor where the work was done. The goal was to reduce waste or non–value-added work in the system, thus increasing employee satisfaction, quality, and productivity and maintaining low production costs. Through years of trial and error, working with the frontline staff, Taiichi Ohno and his team pioneered the lean production business practice known as TPS, which incorporated the principle of meeting the customer's need through a one-by-one continuous flow process with built-in quality indicators and the elimination of system waste.

Another American influence on Toyota was W. Edwards Deming, the American quality pioneer. He defined a "customer" both internally and externally. "Each person or step in a production line or business process was to be treated as a 'customer' and to be supplied with exactly what was needed, at the exact time needed."[1] This view incorporates Toyota's work ethic of demonstrating respect to those who do the work, thus encouraging them to be successful. Another crucial idea adopted from Deming was "a systematic approach to problem solving," referred to as kaizen or continuous improvement, which was intended to sustain TPS daily and to incorporate the frontline staff in decision making.[1]

In the 1960s, Toyota began sharing its successful business practice with its suppliers, creating a "lean enterprise." It was not until the global recession caused by the oil crisis of 1973 that other manufacturing industries in Japan took notice of Toyota. During this time, Toyota did not suffer the great losses of other companies and was asked by the Japanese government to hold seminars on TPS.[1]

American businesses were not exposed to the Toyota Production System until 1982. This exposure was accomplished through a joint venture decision by Eiji Toyoda (chairman) and Shoichiro Toyoda (president) and General Motors, establishing the New United Motor Manufacturing in Fremont, California.[1] Toyota's intention was freely and honestly to share TPS with competitors, whom the company openly acknowledged as contributors to the system of lean production. In a meeting in Japan with Philip Caldwell, the head of Ford Motor Company, Eiji Toyoda stated that, "There is no secret to how we learned what we do, Mr. Caldwell. We learned it at the Rouge."[3] To expand Toyota's teachings to United States industries, the Toyota Supplier Support Center was created in 1992 to provide working TPS models to various plants.[1]

The term "lean production" was introduced in the 1990s by the authors of the book *The Machine That Changed the World,* a Massachusetts Institute of Technology Auto Industry Program that documented what Toyota had discovered decades earlier: "shortening lead time by eliminating waste in each step of a process leads to best quality and lowest cost, while improving safety and morale."[1] It had taken Toyota 40 years to develop its model for producing high-quality cars at low cost, with short lead-time and allowance for broad-based production flexibility. Its dominance of the industry has been unmatched by any other automobile company.

HOW DID TOYOTA DO IT?

Over the last 40 years, Toyota has continued to strive toward the elimination of waste—the heart of TPS—by following a one-by-one continuous flow process. The system is designed to highlight problems in real time, where the work is performed, and solve them to root cause. Many companies have tried to implement this systematic approach to problem solving, but most are unsuccessful. Many emulators focus on the tools used in TPS instead of its basic principles. Moreover, our current "blame culture" is not conducive to this type of system redesign and problem solving. We opt to blame a person and tell him or her to "work harder," rather than to determine the root cause of a problem. A problem often is the result of system-design issues and could be produced by anyone performing the same task.

System errors occur in every industry, and it may be the strategy for addressing them that is critical to success. Solving problems to root cause ensures that they will not recur in a given manner in the future. How does Toyota do it? The question of Toyota's success was addressed in an article by Spear and Bowen,[4] "Decoding the DNA of the Toyota Production System." The authors discovered "unspoken rules that give Toyota its competitive edge." They write, "The system grew naturally out of the workings of the company over five decades . . . it has never been written down and Toyota's workers often are not able to articulate it."[4]

The connection between people and their work is crucial to the success of this process. Leadership support and the involvement of the frontline employee are integral parts of lean production. Spears and Bowen define these connections as the "Four Rules." The first three rules emphasize the design of work. "Rule #1: All work should be highly specified as to content, sequence, timing and outcome. Rule #2: Every customer–supplier connection must be direct and there must be an unambiguous yes-or-no way to send requests and receive responses. Rule #3: The pathway for every product and service must be simple and direct."[4] Rule #4 of the "Four Rules" stresses improvement: "Any improvements must be made in accordance with the scientific method, under the guidance of a teacher, at the lowest possible level in the organization."[4]

Also integral to the TPS model is that "all the rules require that activities, connections, and flow paths have built-in tests to signal problems automatically. It is the continual response to problems that makes this seemingly rigid system so flexible and adaptable to changing circumstances."[4] In Toyota plants, employees are encouraged to announce problems to a team leader by pulling an andon cord, which signals by sound and color where a problem is; acknowledging problems creates the opportunity for improvement. By "lowering the water level in the river to expose all the rocks, [one can] chip away at all the problems."[2] The team leader is used as a real-time problem-solving resource, with one team leader assigned to every four to five team members. On average, an employee pulls the andon cord 12 times per shift.[5] When the team leader solves the problem, the assembly line continues. The line is stopped when the problem cannot be immediately resolved. The problem is then investigated by using the "five whys" to solve it to its root cause. By contrast, our culture traditionally creates "work-arounds" that allow work to continue but do not identify or fully investigate the problem. As a result, problems tend to recur.

A recent book by Jeffrey K. Liker, *The Toyota Way: 14 Management Principles from the World's Greatest Manufacturer,* expands on the success of TPS. "TPS is the most systematic and highly developed example of what the principles of the Toyota Way can accomplish. The Toyota Way consists of the foundational principles of the Toyota culture, which allow TPS to function so effectively."[1] The President of Toyota, Fujio Cho, stated in the 2001 Toyota Way document that "Since Toyota's founding we have adhered to the core principles of contributing to society through the practice of manufacturing high-quality products and services. Our business practices and activities based on this core principle created values, beliefs, and business methods that over the years have become a source of competitive advantage. These are the managerial values and business methods that are known collectively as the Toyota Way."[1]

The Toyota Way is organized into four general categories: "(1) Long-Term Philosophy, (2) The Right Process Will Produce the Right Results, (3) Add Value to the Organization by Developing Your People, and (4) Continuously Solving Root Problems Drives Organizational Learning."[1] The principles associated with each of these categories are listed in Box 1.[1] An examination of these principles clarifies why many companies have been unsuccessful in implementing TPS. Toyota's success is built on its culture of determination, patience, employee involvement, and problem solving by

Box 1. The 14 Toyota Way principles.

Category 1: Long-term philosophy
Principle 1: Base your management decisions on a long-term philosophy, even at the expense of short-term financial goals.

Category 2: The right process will produce the right results
Principle 2: Create continuous process flow to bring problems to the surface.
Principle 3: Use "pull" systems to avoid overproduction.
Principle 4: Level out the workload (heijunka). (Work like the tortoise, not the hare.)
Principle 5: Build a culture of stopping to fix problems, to get quality right the first time.
Principle 6: Standardized tasks are the foundation for continuous improvement and employee empowerment.
Principle 7: Use visual control so no problems are hidden.
Principle 8: Use only reliable, thoroughly tested technology that serves your people and processes.

Category 3: Add value to the organization by developing your people and partners
Principle 9: Grow leaders who thoroughly understand the work, live the philosophy, and teach it to others.
Principle 10: Develop exceptional people and teams who follow your company's philosophy.
Principle 11: Respect your extended network of partners and suppliers by challenging them and helping them improve.

Category 4: Continuously solving root problems drives organizational learning
Principle 12: Go and see for yourself to thoroughly understand the situation (genchi genbutsu).
Principle 13: Make decisions slowly by consensus, thoroughly considering all options; implement decisions rapidly (nemawashi).
Principle 14: Become a learning organization through relentless reflection (hansei) and continuous improvement (kaizen).

Adapted from J. K. Liker, The Toyota Way: 14 Management Principles from the World's Greatest Manufacturer (New York: McGraw-Hill, 2004): 37–41.

the scientific method. Many other industries are unable to commit to long-term plans and lack the resources for root cause problem solving; hence they tend to adopt specific tools of TPS and not the entire system.

CAN "LEAN" HELP THE HEALTHCARE SYSTEM?

The rising costs, decreasing reimbursements, malpractice suits, and shortage and dissatisfaction of healthcare professionals have all contributed to the troubling state of our healthcare system. Questions about the quality of healthcare were brought to the forefront by the staggering statistics in the Institute of Medicine's (IOM) report "To Err Is Human: Building a Safer Health System."[6] The IOM found medical errors (defined as the failure of a planned action to be completed or use of the wrong plan to achieve an aim) to be the "eighth leading cause of death," surpassing deaths from motor vehicle accidents, breast cancer, and AIDS.

In Pittsburgh, there has been a growing initiative to address medical errors. The Pittsburgh Regional Health Care Initiative (PRHI) was formed in 1997 to address the economic and patient safety issues of healthcare in southwestern Pennsylvania, where "healthcare is the largest economic sector, employing one in eight workers and conducting more than $7.2 billion in business."[7] Founded by Paul O'Neill, former U.S. Treasury Secretary and Alcoa Chairman, and Karen Wolk Feinstein, PhD, President of the Jewish Healthcare Foundation, with the mission of providing programs aimed at perfect patient care, PRHI is an alliance of "hundreds of clinicians, 42 hospitals, four major insurers, dozens of major and small business healthcare purchasers, corporate and civic leaders, and elected officials."[7] The Initiative's "patient-centered goals include zero medication errors, zero healthcare-acquired (nosocomial) infections, [and] perfect clinical outcomes, as measured by complications, readmissions, and other patient outcomes, specifically in coronary artery bypass graft surgery and chronic conditions (depression and diabetes)."[7] To accomplish these goals, PRHI has incorporated principles from industrial lean production models, including TPS and

Pittsburgh's Alcoa Business System, to design a model for healthcare called the Perfecting Patient Care (PPC) System.[8] The fundamental principles of the organization are "respect and dignity for everyone, the opportunity for healthcare workers to succeed in doing meaningful work and to have it acknowledged, neutral collaboration among all stakeholders, and improvement based on scientific methods, applied to every patient every day."[7] PRHI offers year-round courses to the public to teach and share the knowledge of the PPC System within the region.

Through grants from the Jewish Healthcare Foundation, the Agency for Health Care Research and Quality, and the University of Pittsburgh School of Medicine, the authors' pathology laboratory chose to adopt the principles of lean production (or the PPC System) to address pathology errors. The implementation of a lean production method begins with leadership support. Leadership throughout the organization, from top administration to frontline supervision, needs to understand and demonstrate approval for the process. Otherwise, implementation will most likely fail. In the authors' organization, implementation began in September 2003 when the laboratory obtained support from the hospital CEO, vice presidents, president, and vice president of the medical staff and developed an education plan for the pathology administration and staff. Education methods included both in-house training sessions and attendance of sessions taught by the PRHI.

Initially, these teachings may be difficult to apply to healthcare because they have manufacturing biases whose relevance may not be apparent. The natural and immediate reaction from some of our laboratory staff was resistance: "We don't make cars here. We work with patient specimens." Several were concerned about the comparison of their work to an industrial process, feeling as if it diminished or simplified their jobs. "You can't apply [the model of] a manufacturing company to our work. Our work is more complicated." Other staff members liked the idea of eliminating waste and improving their work but had doubts that principles from manufacturing could be the answer. Still others expressed their frustration with the current state of the healthcare system and welcomed the idea of trying "anything new" and the opportunity to be part of the change. Everyone wants to take pride in his or her work and achieve success.

ANATOMIC PATHOLOGY LEARNING LINE

To begin establishing what is referred to as a learning line for implementation of a lean production method, one must document the current workflow condition. The role of the team leader (real-time problem solver) for a learning line begins immediately. The leader assures the trust and confidence of the staff involved in implementation through daily teachings and by engaging the staff in generating ideas and sharing information about how they do their work. Observation drawings, a pictorial documentation of workflow pathways, are an important tool adopted from the PPC System.[9] Assumptions about how work is done or should be done often differ from reality. By observing how work is actually performed, one may establish a solid baseline from which to begin workflow and process improvements.

The observation process entails several elements, including demonstrating respect for those one observes. PRHI has established the following recommended Observation Guidelines: "(1) Explain what you are observing to the person being observed and that you are interested in learning from them through observation. They are the teachers of the current condition and you will be observing to learn. (2) Try not to be obtrusive and not to modify the process you are trying to observe. (3) Do not ask 'why' and limit questions. These may be asked at the completion of the observation so as not to interfere. (4) At the end of the observation, thank the person you observed."[9] Although the observation process seems straightforward, this may be a difficult exercise to perform. Staff members will naturally feel uncomfortable performing their work when they know someone is watching their every move and perhaps timing them. In the authors' experience, staff often wanted to point out, "This isn't a normal day" or "This is an unusual circumstance" when they believed the observer might gain a negative impression. It is important to demonstrate sensitivity during these sessions. Other staff members were anxious to explain their work in detail, which was helpful in establishing a comfort level.

To convey the team leader's support for staff work improvement, multiple observations were performed and time was spent talking with the frontline staff. Through data collection and observation drawings, the current condition of the authors' anatomic pathology department was documented, beginning with specimen receipt and ending with the generation of a report to clinicians (Figure D.1). A current condition drawing represents the workflow pathway, drawn according to customer/supplier relationships. The connections between the customer making the request (need) and the supplier meeting the need, as well as how the individual worker performs his or her work (activities), define a pathway.

The authors' anatomic pathology pathway is initiated upon receipt of a specimen from one of their customers (operating room, in-house patients, or outpatient clinics) in the gross room. Here the specimen is appropriately accessioned, grossly examined, and sectioned, with the tissue placed in colored plastic cassettes and the cassettes placed in a rack for the overnight tissue processing machines. The gross room is the supplier of the next step in surgical specimen processing, the histology lab. Histology processes the cassettes the following morning by embedding the tissue in wax and cutting thin pieces of tissue to be stained and placed on a glass slide. The histology lab is the supplier of the pathologist, who reviews the slide and provides a diagnosis for transcription. Transcription then becomes the customer of the pathologist, transcribing the report for the ordering physician. The physician is the supplier of the patient, the ultimate customer.

Included in the current condition drawings are problems, designated as inverted clouds, that have occurred or are system designs to be addressed using the principles of lean. Problems may range from ones as simple as a staff member asking a coworker for a pen and having to search for a supply to more serious ones affecting patient care. Identifying problems is a challenging part of this process. As mentioned earlier, medical culture has adopted the practice of "work-arounds," in which we attempt to solve a problem ourselves and, often without realizing it, create additional steps as a Band-Aid to the problem. Because they do not entail investigating the problem to its root cause, these "work-arounds" become a form of waste in the system. However, it is not easy for workers to acknowledge this extra waste and identify it as a problem. This situation provides another example of the role of the team leader. By working daily with the

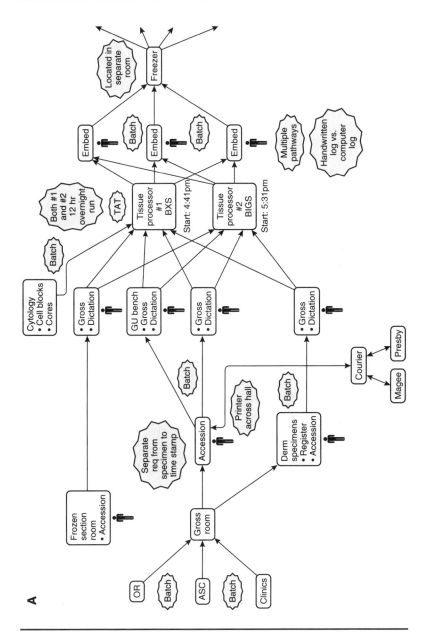

Figure D.1   UPMC Shadyside Anatomic Pathology Laboratory—current condition.

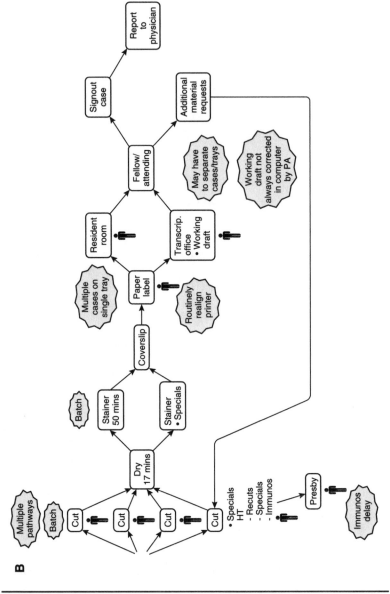

Figure D.1 *Continued.*

staff to teach lean principles and their application to work practices, the leader enables staff to begin identifying the waste in their own work.

Once the current condition has been documented, research focuses on determining the ideal. According to the basic principles of lean, the goals to strive toward are one-by-one and continuous flow work design. Spear and Bowen[4] describe "the notion of the ideal" as essential to understanding TPS. The response to customer need must embody six characteristics: on demand, defect-free, one-by-one, waste-free, immediate, and safe (physically, emotionally, professionally).[4] In pathology, the ultimate goal is to provide appropriate and accurate information about a patient's specimen to a clinician for quality patient care. Ideally, this is accomplished with zero pathology errors (that is, assignments of a diagnosis that does not represent the true nature of disease or nondisease in a patient, as a result of either interpretive or reporting errors). The idea of zero pathology errors may seem unrealistic, but if we do not continually strive toward this theoretic limit, how will we know what is possible? Human potential is limitless—a philosophy practiced successfully by Toyota. As noted previously, everyone wants to succeed at his or her job, though poor system designs often prevent this success.

Demand data are also collected to enhance understanding of the current condition. Demand data (Tables D.1 and D.2) reflect customer need. The mix, volume, and timing of the demand must be understood first (that is, How much of what is needed when?). The next question is "What does it take to make one to perfection?" Mix and volume refer to the type and amount of work.

Table D.1 Anatomic pathology demand data.

Mix	Volume (%)
Biopsy specimens	13
Skin specimens	24
Surgical ("large") specimens	63

Table D.2 Anatomic pathology demand data.

Timing	
Specimens received from	**Pickup times**
OR	8:00 AM, 10:00 AM, 11:00 AM, 1:00 PM, 2:15 PM
ASC	8:00 AM, 10:00 AM, 11:00 AM, 1:00 PM
Clinics	9:00 AM, 9:20 AM, 10:50 AM, 12:15 PM, 12:30 PM, 2:40 PM

For example, the authors' anatomic pathology laboratory receives specimens from the operating room and various physicians' offices and departments. The types of specimens received and processed include soft tissue, bone, prostate, kidney, breast, biopsies, skin, and cytology cell blocks (63 percent surgical specimens, 24 percent skin specimens, 12 percent biopsy specimens, and one percent cytology cell blocks). Each of these types of specimens requires different work to be performed. Timing refers to the frequency of each type of work. The laboratory has both daily scheduled and unscheduled specimen pickups. Fluctuations in volume of certain types of specimens occur daily or weekly.

Once one has established the current condition through workflow observation, problem identification, and collection of demand data, one may determine the direction and possibilities for improving workflow design. The authors' intention was to establish an anatomic pathology learning line and design a one-by-one continuous flow process. Histology, with its inherent "assembly line" workflow design, was designated as the first section of the department to establish this line. Starting with the central portion of the anatomic pathology pathway, one may affect change at both ends of the pathology process.

Once the decision was made to begin in histology, administrative support from histology supervision and the lead histotechnologist was generated. Staff were presented with the current condition and a plan to apply the principles of lean production to improve workflow design and strive toward zero pathology errors. Concentrated teaching began among the team leader, the TPS teacher, and histology staff. Focused observation documented the specific current condition pathway of histology (Figure D.2). This observation focused on

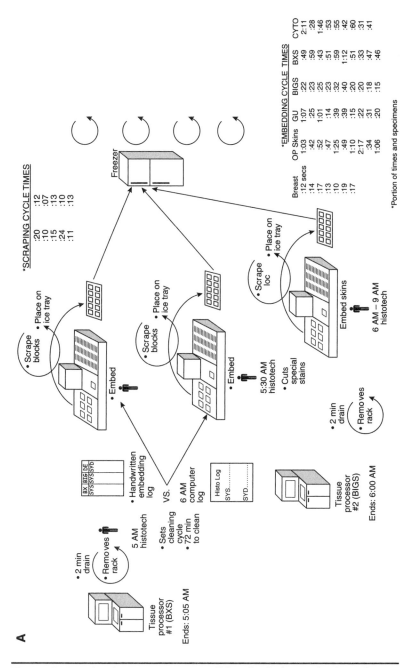

Figure D.2 Histology—current condition (includes cycle times for each task).

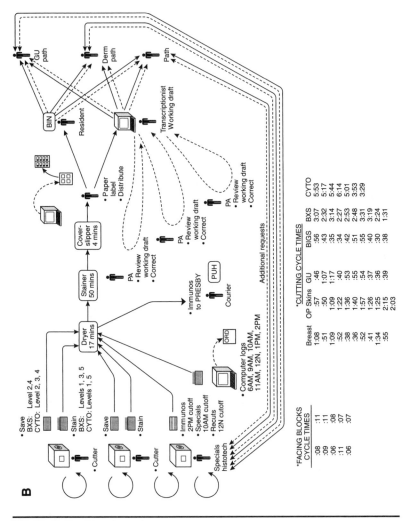

Figure D.2 *Continued.*

how tasks were performed, the amount of time it took to perform each task, how tasks were connected to accomplish work, and problems that arose during the course of work.

Cycle-time data were collected on each histotechnologist for each job task, as was instrumentation timing in the pathway. Cycle time is the time it takes to perform the work activities of one work element (for example, embedding or cutting).[2] For example, the "average" cycle time to embed biopsies was 57 seconds; for cutting, it was 192 seconds, more than triple the amount of time to embed. This discrepancy created an unbalanced workflow, which was evaluated to determine whether any of the cutting tasks could be separated and accomplished at another workstation. For instance, slides could be premade by the embedder to save time for the cutter. This measure is referred to as work balancing, or ensuring that job tasks performed at each station have closer cycle times to maintain balance in the work elements of the pathway. Without work balancing, inventory will build up between work processes. The concept of continuous flow implies that a tissue moves from one work process to the next, with no wasted time waiting in the production line.

Following observational data collection, the histology staff and supervisors of anatomic pathology participated in a lean exercise. Staff were taught the principles of the lean production method through a hands-on exercise in which they mimicked a manufacturing assembly line. The exercise generated mixed reactions from the staff, including resistance to the notion of applying this method to laboratory work, anxiety that the process might eliminate positions, and enthusiasm about trying something different. Leadership was able to address the concerns about position elimination by stressing that this was not the aim of the process.

THE 5S PROCESS

To begin winning the "hearts and minds" of the staff to these new principles, a kaizen—or system improvement—called 5S was initiated. The objective of this process was to clean up and improve the work environment. The process began with a red-tagging session in which the staff placed a red label on any products or equipment they no longer used. All red-tagged items were removed from the laboratory, and the staff decided whether items could be sold, given to another department, or discarded (Figure D.3). The histotechnologists enjoyed this process, because they had wanted to "get rid of the junk" but had not had time to do so. Once the excess was removed, determinations regarding workflow improvements were made using 5S. "5S" refers to the different steps of this process: sort (Japanese seiri, meaning to organize); set in order (seiton, orderliness); shine

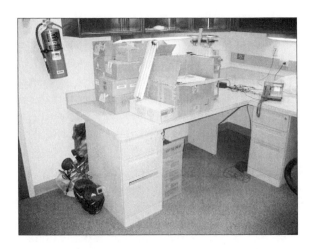

Figure D.3   Portion of items from red-tagging for 5S.

(seiso, cleanliness); standardize (seiketsu, standardized cleanup); and sustain (shitsuke, discipline to maintain this process).[9] To demonstrate the effectiveness of this process, one particular "cell" of the laboratory, the special stain section (Figure D.4), was targeted for redesign, so that only products, supplies, and equipment needed to perform these stains were in the cell.

On one evening, a team consisting of nine members from PRHI, the Clinical Design Team of Shadyside Hospital (which began using the PPC System in 1998 for patient care improvements), the chief and director of Shadyside Pathology, the team leader, the TPS teacher, and additional pathology supervisory staff cleaned the histology laboratory from top to bottom (Figure D.5). From scouring sinks to scrubbing floors and drawers, the team successfully "5S'ed" the laboratory and began creating a visual management atmosphere by tagging drawers to indicate where products were stored (Figure D.6). The next morning, the histotechnologists were pleasantly surprised by the appearance of their lab and the show of support from the staff who accomplished it.

Additional visual management improvements were made in the designated special stain cell by the histotechnologists. These included labeling the outside of the stain and dye cabinets with both

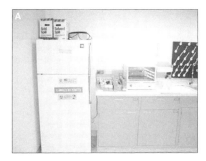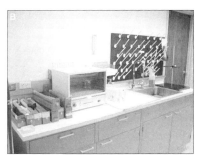
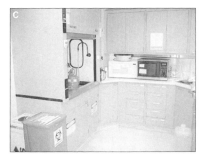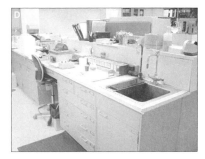

Figure D.4   (*A–D*) Special staining cell before 5S.

pictures and terms to represent what was on the shelf directly behind the cabinet door and color-coding the special stain baskets according to end-color result of each stain (Figure D.7).

During this time, process improvements were also made to address the excess inventory in histology. The histotechnologist responsible for the routine ordering process was instrumental in designing a new replenishment system. This design was accomplished through the use of kanban cards, adopted from TPS.[2] Each product was tagged with a kanban card that included all the information necessary to reorder it: product name, reorder quantity, and trigger point. The trigger point indicated where the card needed to be placed when the product was restocked. This point was determined by calculating the amount of product routinely used and how many days from the ordering date it took to receive the product. The system was based on the three different ordering processes of the laboratory. Products with blue cards, for example, were to be ordered

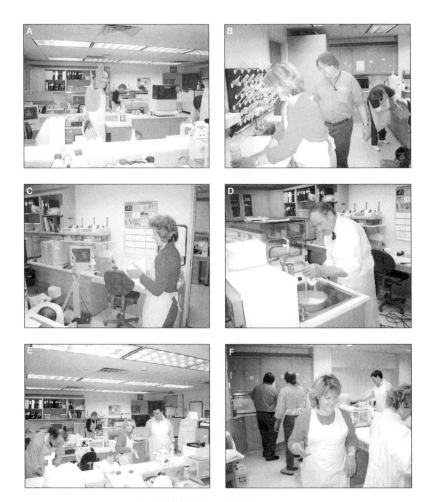

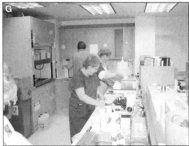

Figure D.5   *(A–G)* 5S group process.

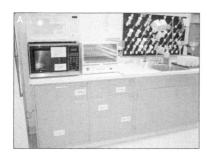
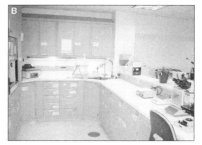

Figure D.6   (*A,B*) Special staining cell after 5S.

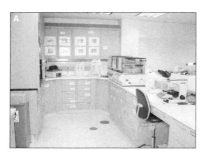
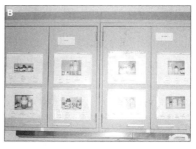
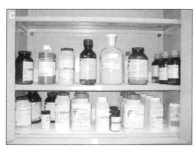
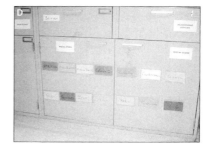
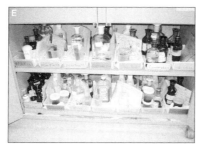

Figure D.7   (*A–E*) Visual management examples.

through a specific vendor, yellow cards were for in-house stock inventory, and pink cards were for the laboratory ordering system. The cards were placed on the product in such a manner as to alert the histotechnologist that it needed to be reordered. When a kanban card was pulled, it was hung on a hook with the corresponding color. It was easy for the histotechnologist to visualize the necessary type of ordering. Once the product was ordered, the card was placed in its corresponding colored bin in the laboratory where products were delivered, so that it could be replaced (Figure D.8). For the ordering histotechnologist, this was a rewarding experience. Her ordering time was cut by at least 50 percent, and she did not have to worry about stocking out or about products not being ordered because someone did not inform her. The system is working well, and the histology laboratory's overstocked inventory has been reduced by approximately 40 percent to 60 percent.

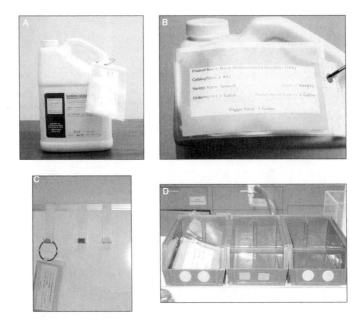

Figure D.8   (*A–D*) Inventory replenishment system (kanban cards). ([A] Courtesy of Anatech Ltd., Battle Creek, Michigan; with permission.)

CONTINUOUS FLOW

The next phase of the authors' implementation was to create a continuous workflow. To create this type of work practice, one must eliminate waste or non-value-added work. Taiichi Ohno[2] describes seven different forms of waste: overproduction, excess movement, excess waiting time, excess inventory, processing waste, transportation waste, and manufacture of defective products. In the laboratory, there are many examples of these forms of waste. For example, laboratory personnel are accustomed to working with large batch sizes, working separately from the next workstation in the process, and having excess inventory on hand.

The waste arising from batching and separation of the different workstations needed to accomplish a process was apparent in the authors' histology department. The original layout of the histology laboratory was as follows: a side room contained three machines for the embedding of tissue and a separate room with five microtomes for the cutting of tissue (Figure D.9). Up to three histotechnologists could be performing the task of embedding at once, while one histotechnologist began cutting. Because the embedders supplied the large number of blocks to be cut, it was necessary to place the blocks on an ice tray in a freezer to keep them cold until a cutter could get to them. This procedure created a large batch of trays for the cutting process. The embedders would pursue their work to completion, then assist with the cutting process. This practice of mass-producing one task, then moving to the next is not unusual and has most likely been practiced for years in many histology laboratories. It does, however, highlight the opportunity to use lean production practices to eliminate these types of system-design waste and to improve pathology practice. When one designs a continuous flow process, one establishes a direct connection between work tasks: the embedder becomes the supplier to the customer, the cutter. To create this direct line of communication in the authors' laboratory, an embedding machine was moved to a counter in the cutting area, and the remainder of the process (primarily instrumentation) was rearranged in order of operation. The end result was a "U-shaped" cell (Figure D.10). This arrangement was a dramatic change for the histotechnologists, who naturally doubted that it would work. The fact that they were willing

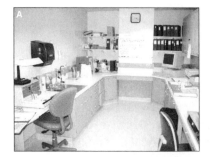
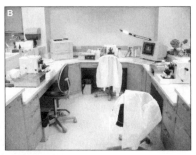

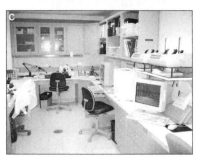

Figure D.9 Histology department layout. (*A*) Embedding room. (*B,C*) Cutting areas.

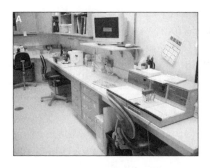
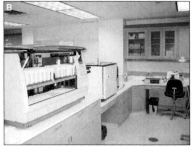

Figure D.10 (*A,B*) Continuous flow.

to try and did not completely resist this experiment in the lean principles was a critical step in the implementation process.

Once the new cell was created, reducing the batch sizes to create a continuous flow and to help prevent the potential for error became an objective. Although the cell had been physically arranged in a continuous flow design, the tendency of the histotechnologists was still to batch-produce at each workstation. Defining and designing the necessary direct connection between the embedder and the cutter required the input of the histotechnologists, those who do the work, under the guidance of the team leader and teacher using the principles of lean. The ideas of not batch-processing and of handing work directly to the cutter (rather than putting trays in the freezer) were significant challenges, because this was unlike any practice the histotechnologists had experienced.

The process began with small experiments intended to demonstrate the true nature of how work is done: one by one; one block, one slide at a time. Answering the question "What is one?" was also challenging. In the gross room, for instance, "one" most likely refers to one patient or one accession number, which could have multiple specimens. In histology, work is performed on tissue blocks to produce slides. When the team had examined the work done on each type of specimen processed, the answer to "What is one?" became a slide. From this determination, it was decided that a maximum of 20 slides (the number that completely filled a slide rack) would be made by the cutter, then passed through the remainder of the process. (This number was chosen for practicality, because of the instrumentation limitation of the stainer.) Hence the embedder (supplier) would send at one time to the cutter (customer) only enough blocks to produce a maximum of 20 slides. This limitation dramatically changed the embedder's work practice. The histotechnologists were being asked to embed only a designated number of blocks—then, once those blocks were appropriately cold, to stop embedding, scrape them, and pass them to the cutter. The cutter previously took her work from the freezer; her work consisted of an ice tray full of blocks, and she filled multiple slide racks before moving them through the process.

Table D.3 illustrates this application of lean production to the reduction of batch sizes, eventually to one, by explaining the amount of work performed on each specimen type. For biopsy specimens,

Table D.3   Histology specimen requirements.

Specimen	No. of slides made	No. of slides stained	No. of slides saved
Biopsy specimens	5	3	2
Cytology cell block	5	2	3
Skin specimens	2	2	0
Surgical ("large") specimens	1	1	0

five slides are made, three are stained, and two are saved for future additional stain requests. These figures mean that the embedder makes and passes six biopsy blocks to the cutter, who makes a total of 18 slides, then sends the slide rack to the dryer to continue the process. If the blocks are from skin specimens, 10 blocks can be made for the cutter to produce 20 slides, and if the blocks are from "large" specimens (for example, tissue sections from a mastectomy), 20 blocks make 20 slides. After many experiments over time, the histotechnologists began developing a comfort level with this new type of production. The work was still not at the ideal state of continuous flow, in which one specimen was embedded at a time and passed directly to the cutter, who made the appropriate number of slides and passed them through the rest of the process. The histotechnologists were, however, able to appreciate that overproduction was not making their work easier or faster; indeed, it had added more stress.

Another important aspect of winning the "hearts and minds" of the staff involved in this lean process was enabling them to recognize the importance of their work. Everyone wants to be successful in his or her job, but often workers are so far removed from their customer that they lack this sense of accomplishment. Pathology is a good example. The diagnosis provided to the clinician by the pathologist has a direct impact on a patient's care. Many are not aware of the complex process needed to provide the most accurate information to the physician. To help bring this end result of their work into perspective for the histotechnologists, a connection was made directly to the patient. The difference was in the thinking: a block is a patient, and work should be performed on that patient continuously to provide an "answer" to him or her as rapidly as possible. To highlight this principle, a bladder specimen was followed through the pathology pathway from its removal from the patient in the operating room to the autofaxing of a report to the physician (Figure D.11). The amount of work actually performed on the specimen (indicated by slashes) was approximately 14 hours, whereas the amount of time the specimen was at rest (open spaces) was approximately 87 hours, including the weekend. This is not unusual pathology practice, and it demonstrates the need to improve our system to decrease the time between collection of a patient specimen and rendering of a diagnosis.

The histotechnologists have demonstrated many successes of adopting a lean process; however, there are still many challenges ahead. As histology approaches the ideal, changes will need to occur at both ends of the pathology pathway. The gross room, for example, should consistently produce tissue blocks with only the amount of (defect-free) tissue necessary for histology to perform its work. Pathologists should be able to sign out cases continuously as they are being produced from histology. At this point, the improvements in the histology pathway have not made significant changes in the overall report turnaround time, but once the gross room and pathology sign-out work elements are incorporated, the authors expect that this time will be significantly reduced.

Currently, the histotechnologists have adopted the practice of smaller batch sizes and continue to work on a true one-by-one processing system. Effective problem solving to root cause will assist in reaching this goal. Once a problem is identified, the team leader and staff work together to identify its cause and find a resolution. PRHI teaches the use of a tool called a Problem Solving A3 (named for the size of paper used to document the problem) to help guide this process.[9] The paper is divided into four quadrants: (1) the background of the process and problem that arose, (2) answers to the "five whys" to determine the root cause of the problem, (3) determination of the target condition in which the problem does not recur, and (4) the action plan or experiments using the scientific method that clearly define the who, what, when, where, and how of the experiment (Table D.4). The authors' histology lab recently encountered a problem that

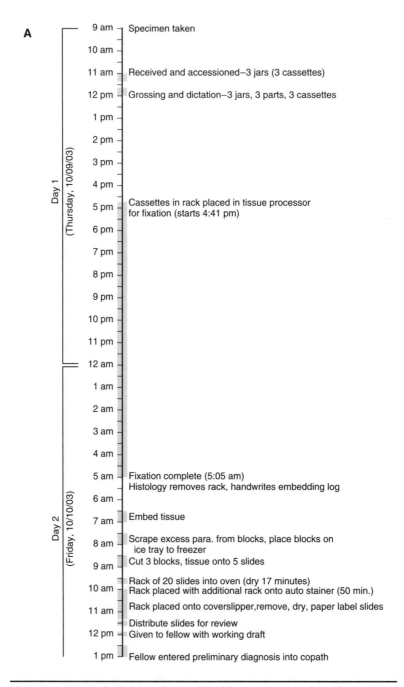

Figure D.11 Pathology pathway: bladder specimen example. *(Continued)*

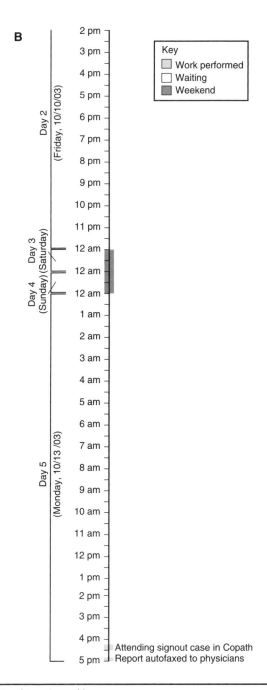

Figure D.11   *(Continued.)*

Table D.4   Problem solving A3.

(1) Background; current condition	(3) Target condition
(2) Problem defined	(4) Action plan

Adapted from Pittsburgh Regional Healthcare Initiative. Perfecting Patient Care System educational materials.

clearly demonstrated the value of solving to the root cause, rather than accepting a superficial solution.

One day, the histotechnologist responsible for cutting slides for immunohistochemistry studies received a computer-generated block order for recuts and additional slides. When she retrieved the block, she noted a scant amount of tissue remaining and observed the number three written on the side of the cassette, indicating the number of pieces originally embedded in the block. She made a notation on the order sheet, "Block very thin before cut immunos," and proceeded to complete the order. Two days later, she received the same request as before, this time with a notation by the pathologist: "*Wrong* block cut!!!" Concerned about and upset by this possible error, the histotechnologist repulled the block and alerted a coworker to the problem. Much time was spent examining other blocks in consecutive order to try to determine how the original slides looked so different from the reprocessed slides. A solution was not determined until later in the day, when the coworker assisting on the case happened to remember a block that had "chunked out" on her microtome a few days earlier. When this accident occurred, the coworker retrieved the remaining specimen from her water bath; thus tissue was available that matched the original slides reviewed by the pathologist. Until this point, the immunohistochemical histotechnologist did not have resolution, and she indicated that she felt "her professionalism was being called into question."

The cause of the scant amount of tissue in the block was actually an instrumentation problem. By standard design, there are two latches in close proximity to each other on the microtome: one to unlock and replace the cutting blade and one to adjust the cutting angle (Figure D.12). On the day of the incident, the histotechnologist had changed her blade and was unaware that the latch for the

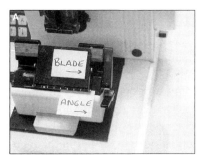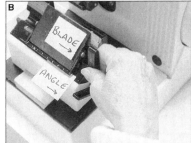

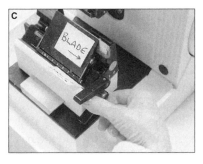

Figure D.12   (*A–C*) Example of root cause analysis. Close proximity of latches enables blade angle to change from routine cutting angle of 10° to 0°.

blade angle had shifted. When she resumed cutting, the blade made a deep cut, resulting in the loss of tissue. Measures are currently being taken to help prevent this from happening again. A rubber stopper is being placed between the two latches to reduce the likelihood of displacing the blade angle.

This story highlights many of the problems we face in healthcare. Had this problem not been solved to its true root cause, the mechanical problem might not have been addressed, and any of the histotechnologists using that microtome could have had the same unfortunate accident. The pathologist, as well as the immunohistochemical histotechnologist herself, would have questioned her professionalism in the future. The pathologist's statement "*Wrong* block cut!!!" immediately created a defensive atmosphere. Placing the blame on a person may be detrimental to finding a solution and, ultimately, to improving the system.

SUMMARY

The current state of our healthcare system calls for dramatic changes. In their pathology department, the authors believe these changes may be accomplished by accepting the long-term commitment of applying a lean production system. The ideal state of zero pathology errors is one that should be pursued by consistently asking, "Why can't we?" The philosophy of lean production systems began in the manufacturing industry: "All we are doing is looking at the time from the moment the customer gives us an order to the point when we collect the cash. And we are reducing that time line by removing non-value-added wastes."[2] The ultimate goals in pathology and overall health care are not so different. The authors' intention is to provide the patient (customer) with the most accurate diagnostic information in a timely and efficient manner. Their lead histotechnologist recently summarized this philosophy: she indicated that she felt she could sleep better at night knowing she truly did the best job she could. Her chances of making an error (in cutting or labeling) were dramatically decreased in the one-by-one continuous flow work process compared with previous practices. By designing a system that enables employees to be successful in meeting customer demand, and by empowering the frontline staff in the development and problem-solving processes, one can meet the challenges of eliminating waste and build an improved, efficient system.

Notes

Chapter 1

1. See "Hospital Bills Spin Out of Control" at http://usatoday.com/
   money/industries/health/2004-04-13-rising-hospital-costs_x.htm,
   http://www.usatoday.com/money/industries/health/
   2003-09-09-healthcare-costs_x.htm, and
   http://www.hospitalconnect.com/hret/publications/content/
   NewRelease.pdf.
2. William J. Latzko and David M. Saunders, *Four Days with
   Dr. Deming* (Reading, MA: Addison Wesley, 1995): 131.
3. See http://www.uaw.org/barg/03/barg02.cfm.
4. See http://www.aier.org/2004pubs/RR01.pdf, "American Institute for
   Economic Research," *Research Reports* 71, no. 1 (2004).
5. Lucette Lagnado, "California Hospitals Open Book, Showing Huge
   Price Differences," *Wall Street Journal* (December 27, 2004):
   A1 and A6. Also available at http://www.trinity.edu/eschumac/
   HCAI5313/WSJ_com%20-%20California%20Hospitals%20Open
   %20Books,%20Showing%20Huge%20Price%20Differences.htm or
   http://suttercorporatewatch.org/news/WSJ12-27-04.pdf.
6. You may read this enlightening report at:
   http://s57.advocateoffice.com/vertical/Sites/%7B56490583-267C-
   4278-BC56-A7128CE248A8%7D/uploads/%7B374CBAD9-740D-
   48BC-8536-92ECD76D1444%7D.PDF
7. See http://jec.senate.gov/democrats/Documents/Reports/
   healthinsurance26aug2004.pdf.

8. David U. Himmelstein, Elizabeth Warren, Deborah Thorne, and Steffie Woolhandler, "Illness and Injury As Contributors to Bankruptcy," *Health Affairs* (February 2, 2005).

9. Melissa Jacoby et. al., "Rethinking the Debates over Health Care Financing: Evidence from the Bankruptcy Courts," *New York University Law Review* 76, no. 2 (May 2001).

10. U.S. Department of Labor Statistics, "Occupational Employment Projections to 2010," *Monthly Labor Review* (November 2001).

11. See http://www.commerce.gov/DOC_MFG_Report_Complete.pdf.

12. See www.Lean.org.

13. James Womack and Dan Jones, *Lean Thinking* (New York: Simon & Schuster, 1996).

14. Steffie Woolhandler, MD, "Cost of Health Care Administration in the United States and Canada," *New England Journal of Medicine* 349, no. 8 (August 21, 2003): 768–75.

15. For an in-depth discussion of administrative costs and waste, see http://www.citizen.org/publications/release.cfm?ID=7271. This site also contains a good discussion of the advantages of single-payer systems such as the Canadian healthcare system.

16. See http://www.cms.hhs.gov.

17. See http://www.who.int.

18. See http://www.intelihealth.com/IH/ihtIH/WSMST000/333/8896/377730.html.

19. Gerard Anderson, "Comparing Health System Performance in OECD Countries," *Health Affairs* 20, no. 3 (May/June 2001): 219–32.

20. The most recent complete comparative data analyses for infant mortality rates are from 1996, according to the National Center for Health Statistics "Preventing Infant Mortality," HHS Fact Sheet, U.S. Department of Health and Human Services, April 8, 2000.

21. See http://www.mbgh.org.

22. See http://www.ripolicyanalysis.org/QualityofCareinUS.pdf or www.nejm.org.

23. Robin E. McDermott, *The Basics of FMEA* (Portland, OR: Productivity Press, 1996).

24. See http://www.programbusiness.com/NewsFinance/ArticleDetail.asp?artID=1372 and http://www.usatoday.com/money/industries/health/2004-04-12-hospital-coverside_x.htm.

25. For another good presentation of how to monitor community health status indicators, see http://www.doh.state.fl.us/family/mch/docs/fy2003/fy2003support1.pdf.

Chapter 3

1. For discussions of payer and financing systems and macro healthcare delivery issues, you may refer to John P. Geyman, "The Corporate Transformation of Medicine and Its Impact on Costs and Access to Care" *Journal of the American Board of Family Practice* 16, no. 5 (September–October 2003): 443–54 at http://www.jabfp.org/cgi/content/full/16/5/443 or to articles by Marcia Angell or George D. Lundberg, *Severed Trust* (New York: Basic Books, 2000).

2. For an example of how nationally the recognized SSM Healthcare of St. Louis, MO, uses a graphical method to monitor key indicators, see section seven of their winning Baldrige National Quality Award application at http://baldrige.nist.gov/PDF_files/SSM_Application_Summary.pdf. Another graphical scorecard example from Saint Luke's Hospital of Kansas City, MO, may be seen in section 7 at http://www.mqa.org/pdf/SLHcat7.pdf. St. Luke's is the first healthcare organization to win the prestigious Missouri Quality Award and has since become the first three-time recipient of it.

3. Taiichi Ohno, *Toyota Production System: Beyond Large-Scale Production* (Cambridge, MA: Productivity Press, 1988): 41.

4. Christine Tierney, "Big 3 Still Lagging Japan," *Detroit News* (February 22, 2004)

5. See "To Fix Health Care, Hospitals Take Tips from Factory Floor," *Wall Street Journal* (April 9, 2004) at http://www.ihaonline.org/frimailing/2004/$_{2004}$%20Enclosures/NS4-9-04.pdf.

6. James Womack, *The Machine That Changed the World: The Story of Lean Production* (New York: Harper Perennial, 1991): 62.

7. Ibid, p. 81.

8. Kiyoshi Suzaki, *The New Manufacturing Challenge: Techniques for Continuous Improvement* (New York: The Free Press, 1987): 17.

9. Neil Swideg, "The Revolutionary," *Boston Globe Magazine* (January 4, 2004).

10. *Technology Law Newsletter* (Spring 2003), available at www.computerbar.org.

11. See www.websense.com and its competitors.

12. Ohno, *Toyota Production*, 130.

13. See http://news.yahoo.com/news?tmpl=story&u=/ap/20040604/ap_on_he_me/doctor_visits_1.

14. To learn more, please see http://baldrige.nist.gov/index.html and http://www.nist.gov/public_affairs/releases/ssmhealth.htm and http://www.ssmhc.com/internet/home/ssmcorp.nsf.

15. See http://www.ebaptisthealthcare.org/BaptistHospital/ and http://www.startribune.com/stories/308/4014401.html.

Chapter 5

1. See http://www.unitedwaymc.org/media/LIFE-Health.pdf.

Appendix D

Reprinted from *Clinics in Laboratory Medicine,* 24(4), Condel, Sharbaugh, and Raab, "Error-Free Pathology: Apply Lean Methods to Anatomic Pathology," pp. 865–99, copyright 2004, with permission from Elsevier.

1. J. Liker, *The Toyota Way: 14 Management Principles from the World's Greatest Manufacturer* (New York: McGraw-Hill, 2004).
2. T. Ohno, *Toyota Production System: Beyond Large-Scale Production* (Cambridge, MA: Productivity Press, 1988).
3. H. Johnson and A. Broms, *Profit Beyond Measure: Extraordinary Results Through Attention to Work and People* (New York: The Free Press, 2000).
4. S. Spear and K. Bowen, *Decoding the DNA of the Toyota Production System* (Harvard Business Press, 1999).
5. K. Mishina and K. Takeda, *Toyota Motor Manufacturing, USA, Inc.* (Harvard Business School, 1992).
6. Institute of Medicine, *To Err Is Human: Building a Safer Health System* (Washington, DC: National Academy Press, 1999).
7. Pittsburgh Regional Healthcare Initiative Web site. Available at: www.prhi.org. Accessed March 2004.
8. K. Feinstein, N. Grunden, and E. Harrison, "A Region Addresses Patient Safety" *American Journal of Infection Control* 30, no. 4 (2002): 248–51.
9. Pittsburgh Regional Healthcare Initiative. *Perfecting Patient Care System Educational Materials* (Pittsburgh: PRHI, 2002).

Bibliography

Berk, Joseph, and Susan Berk. *Total Quality Management: Implementing Continuous Improvement.* New York: Sterling Publishing, 1993.

Bodenstab, Charles J. *A New Era in Inventory Management for the Distribution Industry.* Minneapolis, MN: Hilta Press, 1993.

Carey, Raymond G. *Measuring Quality Improvement in Healthcare—A Guide to Statistical Process Control Applications.* New York: Quality Resources, 1995.

Crosby, Philip B. *Quality Is Free: The Art of Making Quality Certain.* New York: Mentor, 1980.

Dillon, Andrew P., trans. *The Sayings of Shigeo Shingo: Key Strategies for Plant Improvement.* Cambridge, MA: Productivity Press, 1985.

Dobyns, Lloyd. *Thinking About Quality: Progress, Wisdom, and the Deming Philosophy.* New York: Times Books, Random House, 1994.

Feld, William M. *Lean Manufacturing Tools, Techniques, and How to Use Them.* Boca Raton, FL: The St. Lucie Press, 2001.

Fisher, Dennis. *The Just-in-Time Self Test.* Chicago: Irwin Professional Publishing, 1995.

George, Michael L. *Lean Six Sigma for Service.* New York: McGraw-Hill, 2003.

Gross, John M. *Kanban Made Simple.* New York: AMACOM American Management Association, 2003.

Henderson, Bruce A. *Lean Transformation: How to Change Your Business into a Lean Enterprise.* Richmond, VA: The Oaklea Press, 1999.

Hines, Peter. *Value Stream Management.* Harlow, England and Reading, MA: Prentice Hall, 2000.

Hirano, Hiroyuki. *5S for Operators: 5 Pillars of the Visual Workplace.* Portland, OR: Productivity Press, 1996.

Japan Management Association. *Kanban: Just-in-Time at Toyota.* Portland, OR: Productivity Press, 1985.

Johnson, H. *Profit Beyond Measure: Extraordinary Results through Attention to Work and People.* New York: The Free Press, 2000.

Kobayashi, Iwao. *20 Keys to Workplace Improvement.* Cambridge, MA: Productivity Press, 1988.

Lamprecht, James L. *ISO 9000: Preparing for Registration.* Milwaukee: ASQC Quality Press, 1992.

Latzko, William J. *Four Days with Dr. Deming.* Reading, MA: Addison-Wesley, 1995.

Liker, Jeffrey K. *The Toyota Way: 14 Management Principles from the World's Greatest Manufacturer.* New York: McGraw-Hill, 2004.

Lundberg, George D., MD. *Severed Trust: Why American Medicine Hasn't Been Fixed.* New York: Basic Books, Perseus Books Group, 2000.

McDermott, Robin E. *The Basics of FMEA: Failure Mode and Effects Analysis.* Portland, OR: Productivity Press, 1996.

Mears, Peter. *Quality Improvement Tools & Techniques.* New York: McGraw-Hill, 1995.

Nauman, Earl, and Steven H. Hoisington. *Customer Centered Six Sigma.* Milwaukee: ASQ Quality Press, 2001.

Ohno, Taiichi. *Toyota Production System: Beyond Large-Scale Production.* Cambridge, MA: Productivity Press, 1988.

Pande, Pete. *What Is Six Sigma?* New York: McGraw-Hill, 2002.

Salvendy, Gavriel, ed. *Handbook of Industrial Engineering.* New York: John Wiley & Sons, 2001.

Sandras, William A. Jr. *Just-in-Time: Making It Happen.* Essex Junction, VT: Oliver Wight Limited Publications, 1989.

Schonberger, Richard J. *Japanese Manufacturing Techniques: Nine Hidden Lessons in Simplicity.* New York: The Free Press, 1982.

Slater, Robert. *29 Leadership Secrets from Jack Welch.* New York: McGraw-Hill, 2003.

Suzaki, Kiyoshi. *The New Manufacturing Challenge: Techniques for Continuous Improvement.* New York: The Free Press, 1987.

———. *The New Shop Floor Management: Empowering People for Continuous Improvement* (New York: The Free Press, 1993.

To Err Is Human: Building a Safer Health System. Washington, DC: National Acedemy Press, 1999.

White House Domestic Policy Council. *The President's Health Security Plan.* New York: Times Books, Random House, 1993.

Womack, James P. *The Machine That Changed the World: The Story of Lean Production.* New York: Harper Perennial, 1991.

Zandin, Kjell B., ed. *Maynard's Industrial Engineering Handbook.* New York: McGraw-Hill, 2001.

Index